CANNABIS
A Big Sisters' Guide

Anna May Meade
Mary Meade

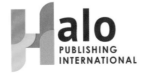

Halo
PUBLISHING
INTERNATIONAL

Graphic Design and Illustration: Erica Giokas
Photography: A. Sullivan
Cover Photo: Bask, Inc.
Back Cover Photos: Bask, Inc, & Beverly Meade

ISBN: 978-1-61244-767-4
Library of Congress Control Number: 2019910024

Printed in the United States of America

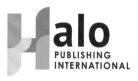

Published by Halo Publishing International
1100 NW Loop 410
Suite 700 - 176
San Antonio, Texas 78213
www.halopublishing.com
contact@halopublishing.com

Disclaimer

Things move fast! We strive to present the most cutting-edge information available at the time of publication. This book contains the authors' personal opinions, insights, and information based on extensive research and anecdotal evidence. The authors of this book are not medical practitioners or attorneys and cannot provide advice in those areas. The laws in the United States and around the world are changing around cannabis. US federal and state laws apply to the use of cannabis in America, so it may not be legal where you are located or if you are traveling between states. Consult with a licensed, experienced attorney prior to making legal decisions (even if it is not our awesome youngest sister). Consult a physician or other health care professional before making any healthcare decisions.

Special Thanks

We are deeply grateful for the overwhelming support and encouragement from all of our family, friends, and helping hands we met along the way. Most of the passionate people in this business have a story, a personal connection to how this plant has transformed their lives. We are pleased to be able to tell some of those stories. Big thanks to the big sisters Aja, Goldie, Mikki, Sarah, and TaShonda; we're happy that we can share your journey.

To all our amazing contributors, thank you for believing in our vision and sharing yours. Accuvape, Hilary Dulany, Bask, Chappie and Joanne, Davinci, Fli, Jeremy, Freedom Leaf, Ray, Goldleaf, Charles ~ so beautiful, Dr. Bonni Goldstein, for your leadership, Green Goddess Supply, The Green Torch, Viondy, Barcelona Hash, Marihuana & Hemp Museum, Thanks Ferenz, The Healing Rose, Laura, Healing Tree Edibles, Mikki and Sarah, High on Love, Angela, Ire CBD, Dan McKeon, MCR Labs, Sana Packaging, S. Richardson, Two Roots, Urban Grow, and Wana Brands.

Thanks Mom, for suggesting I write a book; Dad for who I am; my sisters: Mary for seeing me and reminding me of it, Rose for love and expertise, Chris for love and laughter. Erica and Mandy, thank you for making this fun. And all y'all on my cannabis journey ~ we had some fun. Love ya.

—ANNA

Thank you to my son and coach, Jack Smith IV, for helping me on this cannabis and cancer journey; my sister Anna Meade for sharing everything she knows about the plant; my parents, Beverly and James, for teaching me how to self educate and research; my sisters, Chris Gilman and Rose Meade Hart, for their support on my cancer journey no matter where it leads; Tina Gilman, for all her love and support during this long road to health; my friends, Jack Smith III, Joanne Douds, Kathy Yamaoka, Eva Rassmussen, and Rev. Regina Christianson for being everything that's needed on this most difficult journey. To Erica, for a special introduction to edibles, a whole new world.

—MARY

Table of Contents

ABOUT THIS BOOK

Cannabis, or marijuana, is all over the news. Every year more states and countries are changing their laws to allow medical or adult use of cannabis. But what is cannabis? Is it the same weed people smoked in the 60's? Will it get you high and give you the munchies? Some say it is a miracle drug.

We are here to answer your questions. What is cannabis, how do you get it, how to use it, and why would you want to. So relax, enjoy, and let's get rolling.

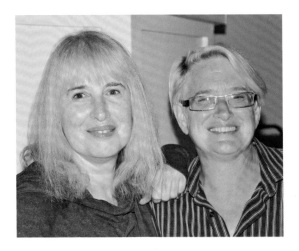

Photo courtesy of Dan McKeon

Mary and Anna are sisters. Like many sisters we share stories and have our different perspectives. We lead very different lives, but when there is a problem, we help each other and figure out how to move forward.

> **Buzz Words**
> **Cannabis:** Weed, pot, marijuana, hash, hemp, ganja, grass, herb; there are many different names for this infamous plant but they all mean the same thing. We mostly use cannabis, as it is the name of the plant and includes all of the species.

Mary's Story

My journey from stage four cancer to cannabis started with pain associated with a non-healing wound. I asked my son, a millennial, what did he know about cannabis? It turns out he had done a lot of research, knew all about his favorites, and how they affected him.

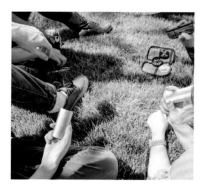

Photo courtesy of Davinci

We went out to lunch with his friends; they all shared their best ideas. I wanted to sleep better without resorting to pain medication. Stage four patients often get prescribed strong medications like morphine. That worked for me but it made me feel dopey all day long, even though I only took it at night. Every other pain med made me feel like I had the flu.

The first time I smoked a bong I had no pain, just a comfortable feeling, then a feeling of wellness. That's something cancer patients rarely feel: wellness.

I wanted to figure out how best to use cannabis: I complained to my son. I needed a coach! He said the problem is people would rather not have a candid conversation because it is illegal in most states. After all, people will tell you not to mix beer and liquor, or where to get the best prices on rosé. There are a lot of choices; bongs, pipes, what's best?

I explored cannabis and discovered I like edibles. A few gummies combined with lower doses of opioids helped me get to sleep and stay asleep. Less pain meds meant less brain fog. Sleeping well was a big part of my recovery from two major surgeries. When I dropped the opioids, I had very small withdrawal symptoms. I took more cannabis,

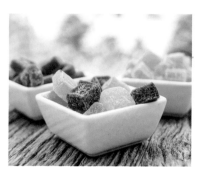

Photo courtesy of Wana Brands

which smoothed out those side effects, headaches, muscle aches, restless leg, and insomnia.

Anna's Story

Through my work as an environmental scientist, I traveled all over the world. I enjoyed this herb in many places. Over the past few decades, our thinking has evolved. In some places, cannabis was decriminalized, allowed for medicinal uses, or legalized for general adult use.

It is known as an ancient herb, used by early Egyptians and is even mentioned in the bible. It was criminalized for political reasons and social justice must be part of the end of prohibition.

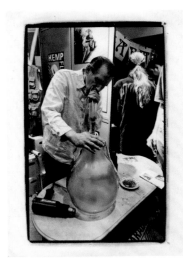

Photo courtesy of the Hash, Marihuana & Hemp Museum

Cannabis Tales: Coffee Shops in Amsterdam

For decades, Amsterdam was the destination for legal weed. Cannabis sales are limited to "coffee shops." They have a separate marijuana menu, with strains of marijuana and hash. You buy your weed and a beverage and you can light up and enjoy. When I visited a coffee house, I met people from all over the world. Several planned an airline layover so they could enjoy a coffee shop. Several gifted me the rest of their purchase, as I was staying for a week. Lucky me.

In May 2015, my sister Mary was diagnosed with Stage 4 breast cancer. It was a difficult few years. Between pain and drug side effects, Mary was having trouble sleeping. She began smoking herb to relax before bed. When a person is very sick, sleep can be the best medicine.

I was happily surprised how much cannabis helped her. She told me: "It helps me relax and get deep restful sleep, which helps healing. In the morning, I wake up clear, without brain fog or exhaustion. If the only thing cannabis did was allow people to get a good night's sleep, it would be amazing. The only side effect is that there is less morning stiffness in my feet."

I have been a cannabis enthusiast for many years. I enjoy cannabis to feel more creative, to de-stress, or just relax with friends. I live in a state that has legalized cannabis and was developing new cannabis businesses. Suddenly, cannabis was also a way I could help my sister.

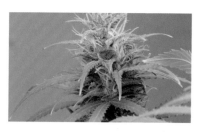

Photo courtesy of S. Richardson

My sisters and I often support and coach each other, so it was natural for us to work together to explore cannabis. The upside of this whole ordeal is that we became much closer.

We realized that many people could benefit from cannabis and might need a coach, but may not have a sister to help them, so we decided to write a book to answer basic questions. Our friends were excited and everyone seems to know someone who could really use this information.

WHAT'S THE BUZZ ABOUT CANNABIS?

What is cannabis? It's like saying what is alcohol; there are different types and brands. Cannabis is a plant. Marijuana, grass, herb, pot, ganja, weed, and hemp are different names for cannabis. What most people are smoking now is called flower. It is the flower or the bud from the mature female cannabis plant.

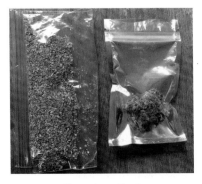

Photo: Anna Meade

In the past people bought a baggie of loosely ground leaves, stems, and seeds that looked vaguely like oregano. You had to clean out the seeds before you smoked it. That is not what people are doing today.

You won't find seeds in the cannabis you buy today. Growers separate the male flowers to prevent the formation of seeds. This encourages the flowers to get larger and more potent. Cannabis was called weed because it is a fast growing herb. Today it is the complete opposite of a weed; it is highly cultivated, regulated, and differentiated.

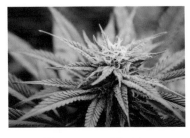

Photo courtesy of Bask Inc

The part of the plant that people are smoking today is the bud, or unpollinated flower, also called sinsemilla. Some leaves around the flower seem to have a sugar coating and are called sugar leaves. The essential oils that give cannabis its effects are concentrated on the bud and sugar leaves.

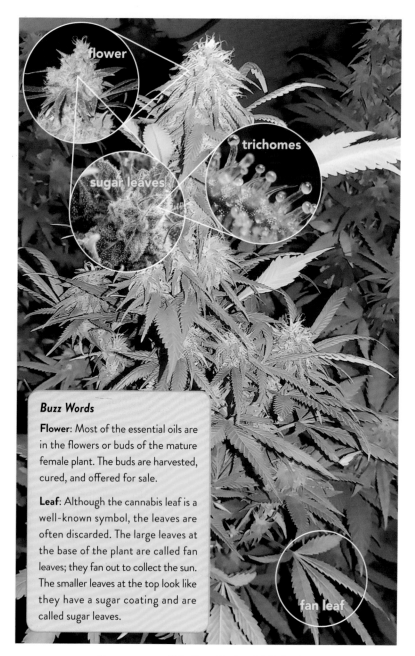

flower

trichomes

sugar leaves

fan leaf

Buzz Words

Flower: Most of the essential oils are in the flowers or buds of the mature female plant. The buds are harvested, cured, and offered for sale.

Leaf: Although the cannabis leaf is a well-known symbol, the leaves are often discarded. The large leaves at the base of the plant are called fan leaves; they fan out to collect the sun. The smaller leaves at the top look like they have a sugar coating and are called sugar leaves.

Photos courtesy of The Green Torch and S. Richardson

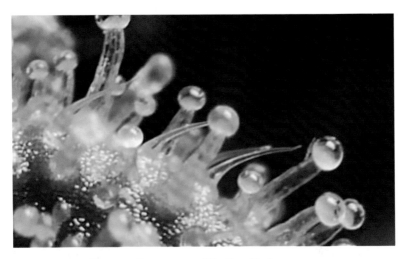

Photo courtesy of The Green Torch

Looking closer, you see the sugar coating is actually a stem with a small drop of essential oil. These stems are called trichomes, and the essential oils are concentrated cannabinoids, terpenes, and flavonoids. While the top of the plant gets most of the attention, the whole plant, even the roots, has medicinal benefits.

Buds are harvested when they are mature. They are carefully dried and cured to preserve their potency. The buds are trimmed and packaged. Batches will be tested before shipment for processing and sales.

Buzz Words

Trim: During harvest, the leaves are cut away from the bud. The cut leaves are called trim. Trim, especially sugar leaves, is often used to make extracts.

Sinsemilla: The buds of the female plant, with a large concentration of the desirable essential oils.

Trichomes: Hairs around the flower that look like sugar frosting. These hairs make resins, or essential oils, that contain cannabinoids, terpenes, and flavonoids, which give each strain its flavor and personality.

Dank: The best buds, sticky with cannabinoids.

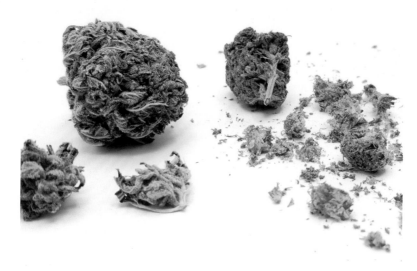

Photo: A. Sullivan

The essential oils, or cannabinoids on the plant, change as the plant develops and is harvested. They change again when the plant is dried and prepared for sale. Heating cannabis also changes it; the molecules get smaller or decarboxylated. This allows them to affect your brain, triggering the signature "high" from THC (tetrahydrocannabinol). A chart in the appendix shows how the cannabinoids change.

When properly dried, cannabis should be a little spongy with its leaves intact. Store it in a dark, airtight container; exposure to light and air dries out your herb. Old cannabis tends to be more of a sedative as the cannabinoids change.

It is not just smoking anymore. There are many ways to consume cannabis. The essential oils can be extracted and infused in foods or heated and inhaled like an electronic cigarette. While brownies are traditional, people are infusing cookies, candies, and savory foods with cannabis.

In addition to smoking and eating cannabis, you can also absorb it through your skin. Tinctures, patches, and creams are available. New products are being developed every day to help people enjoy the benefits of cannabis.

Strains – Different Varieties

Just like there are many different varieties of potatoes, there are different varieties of cannabis, known as strains, or cultivars. Not all cannabis makes you high and gives you the munchies. Different strains have different effects.

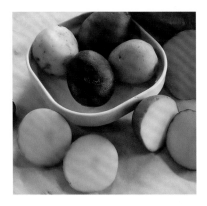

Two varieties of cannabis are sativas and indicas. Different regional climates made them develop differently. People thought each variety would have certain effects.

Photo: A. Sullivan

It was understood that sativas were energizing and euphoric, suitable for daytime. Indicas tended to be relaxing and calming; used for sleep. Both could get you high. We are learning that looking at the terpenes and cannabinoids is a better way to judge how each strain will affect you.

Most strains are hybrids, cross-breeds of indicas and sativas. Growers breed plants to produce certain terpene and cannabinoid profiles. There are hundreds of strains that promise certain effects. However, growing conditions also affect the plant. The same strain may vary from place to place.

Buzz Words

Cannabis Sativa: Taller narrow leaf varieties that thrive in warmer climates. Thought to have stimulating effects.

Cannabis Indica: Shorter broad leaf varieties that thrive in colder climates. Assumed to have sedating effects.

Hemp: Cannabis varieties with minimal THC.

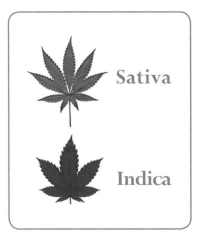

Sativa

Indica

Cannabis Tales: Presidential Crops

George Washington, Thomas Jefferson, and other colonial farmers grew hemp as a cash crop. It was easy to grow and had strong fibers. Washington's diary showed that he also grew Indian Hemp and was interested in its medicinal uses. There is speculation, but no record, of him chewing the leaves to relieve tooth pain.

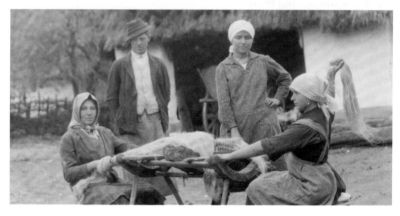

Photo courtesy of Hash Marihuana & Hemp Museum

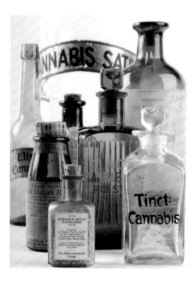

Photo courtesy of Hash Marihuana & Hemp Museum

Cannabis has been cultivated in America since colonial times for medicine and textiles. Cannabis plants have many other uses, such as food, textiles, and building materials. The fibers were used to make clothing, paper, rope, and sails for ships.

The Marijuana Tax Act in 1937 ended widespread medical use and stunted research. Laws were enacted to limit the importation and use of Mexican marijuana and Indian hemp. Imports of hemp from Europe were protected. Industrial hemp plants were bred to have strong fibers.

Later, laws categorized cannabis by the amount of THC in the plant. Hemp, with a minimal amount of THC, was legal. Varieties with a higher THC concentration were designated as marijuana and illegal.

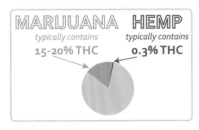

Image: Erica Giokas

Cultivation of cannabis focused on limiting THC for legal hemp or maximizing THC content for the illegal market. Both hemp and marijuana plants produce various cannabinoids and terpenes.

As cannabis is becoming mainstream, more strains and products are being offered. Catchy strain names are good marketing tools. National brands are emerging. Some firms offer a spectrum of products based on the effects: sleep, calm, balance, awaken, or energy, etc.

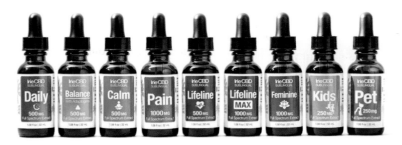

Photo courtesy of Irie CBD

Did you know?

The cannabis plant can draw toxic chemicals from the soil. Industrial hemp was used to remove radiation from the soil around Chernobyl. The roots of the plant draw the chemicals out of the soil and into the plant. Phytoremediation has been used to clean up soil contaminated with heavy metal and industrial pollutants in many places. All cannabis plants pull chemicals from the soils. Make sure your cannabis is tested and grown organically.

SISTERS SAY

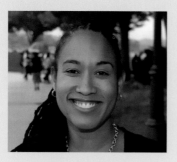

Photo courtesy of TaShonda Vincent-Lee

TaShonda Vincent-Lee
Co-Founder and Director of
Community Outreach, Elevate NE
Community Outreach and Events
Manager, Tilt Holdings

What is your cannabis journey?

It has not been a clear path, but that's life. When I was a sophomore in college, my friends and I decided to try it. I remember thinking "Wow! This is not something I want to try again." It must have been an indica, with a lot of myrcene, which is a sedative. I didn't like the feeling of not having control. My friends agreed. We had one joint and we chucked it.

In my twenties, I was diagnosed with debilitating disorders and prescribed a stimulant & SSRI. These prescription drugs counteracted each other and increased my symptoms. I told my doctor: "I don't like the side effects of my medication. I don't like the way I feel. They helped me to focus, but they weren't helping me emotionally." None of my friends wanted to hang out with me; so I wanted to pursue more holistic medicine.

This time cannabis was a completely different experience. I felt really clear-headed and focused. I felt like myself, just more balanced. My friends and I enjoyed the day shopping and came home. With cannabis, no one could tell I wasn't on my medications. So I decided not to take them on the weekends.

If something made me feel better, then I felt I had a right to try it. I did research and found that it was non-toxic and from 1851 to 1937 was included in the U.S. Pharmacopeia, the doctor's Desk Reference of that time. As I began to understand the industries that benefitted from prohibition, it blew my mind.

Unfortunately, I suffered a tragic loss in 2013. During a session, I disclosed to my therapist that cannabis helped me and I didn't understand why I couldn't simply use cannabis in lieu of narcotic prescriptions. My therapist said, "If we lived in a state where medical marijuana was legal, then you would be a perfect candidate." When I moved to Massachusetts, I made sure that I could use the medication that was best for me. I became a registered Medical Marijuana patient, then an advocate, and now a professional in the industry.

What is your favorite?

I'm an old-fashioned girl. I enjoy a nice joint or a pre-roll. As a medical marijuana patient, I am looking for different terpene and cannabinoid profiles to treat my symptoms. My tolerance level is pretty high, so I often look for a THC profile anywhere between 23-29% in the Massachusetts market. The best strain I've consumed in a very long time was Kalifa Kush, on a trip to Vegas.

What do you want people to know?

I think the biggest misconception is that this is a gateway drug. For me it has been a gateway to health and an exit from my prescription drugs.

CHOOSING CANNABIS

There are many reasons you may want to consider using cannabis. You may have heard that CBD is miracle drug or that THC will get you high. You need to decide what is right for you.

The essential oils in cannabis can help to relieve inflammation and pain. These essential oils are cannabinoids, terpenes, and flavonoids. Terpenes and flavonoids are also found in other plants, but cannabis is the only plant that has cannabinoids.

Did you know?

Your body naturally produces cannabinoids. In fact, mother's milk contains cannabinoids. Researchers are finding that some diseases, like fibromyalgia, may be caused from not having enough cannabinoids in your system!

These essential oils work with your internal systems to balance your body. In fact, all animals have an internal system that uses cannabinoids, called the endo-cannabinoid system or ECS.

Your brain makes things happen in your body via your nervous system. Nerve cells send signals from neurotransmitters to receptors to organs to activate responses. These flow only in one direction and can misfire, causing pain, inflammation, and spasms.

Your ECS helps to keep your body running smoothly by providing signals back to the sending neuron. This is known as retrograde-signaling. Your ECS seeks to keep your body balanced in a state of equilibrium known as homeostasis. Cannabinoids trigger receptors on the neurotransmitters that modify, amplify, or stop the signals. For example, THC reacts with serotonin receptors to relieve depression.

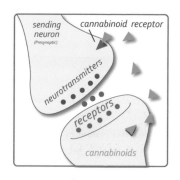

Image: Erica Giokas

There are cannabis receptors in the brain, immune system, and throughout the body. They affect pain, appetite, memory, inflammation, and immune responses.

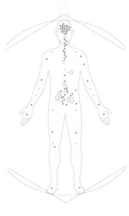

Cannabis acts on receptors in your brain and can help with chronic pain, anxiety, and Post-Traumatic Stress Disorder (PTSD). Cannabis interacts with your immune system and has also been known to provide relief from autoimmune diseases like multiple sclerosis (MS), fibromyalgia, and arthritis.

Each person's system is different. That is why the same cannabis may affect people differently. While a particular type of cannabis may affect many people in one way, you may have a very different experience. Even more, your system also changes due to stress, hormones, and other factors. Herbal medicine is very personal.

Image courtesy of Goldleaf

Did you know?
All animals have an ECS system. Cannabis is understood to affect pets like it does humans. Many products may help our furry friends find relaxation or pain relief. Consult your vet for your pets' overall health. Secure your stash from curious paws and claws to keep your pets safe.

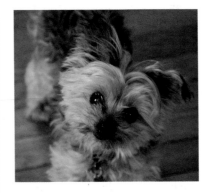

Photo: Anna Meade

What are THC and CBD?

Some think that CBD is the healer and THC is the partier, but THC also has healing properties. Cannabinoids interact with our ECS to create effects like pain relief, inflammation reduction, relaxation, or euphoria. The two most common cannabinoids, CBD and THC, are thought to be the main drivers of the effects.

Other cannabinoids, like CBG and CBN, are often critical. Like baking, your bread won't be the same without a small amount of yeast. For example, a little CBN combined with THC produces a strong sedative. Unlike baking, however, cannabis research is in its infancy.

THC

CBD

Image: Erica Giokas

Generally, THC can alleviate pain and nausea and makes you feel high and hungry. CBD can relieve anxiety, pain, and inflammation and is calming and non-intoxicating. Taken together, they enhance and balance each other. You can group available strains into THC-dominant, CBD-dominant, and balanced THC/CBD strains.

> **Buzz Words**
>
> **THC**: Tetrahydrocannabinol (THC) is a common cannabinoid in cannabis. It gives you the euphoric or high feeling.
>
> **CBD**: Cannabidiol (CBD) does not have intoxicating effects and can balance or counteract the anxiety produced by THC.
>
> **Entourage effect**: Cannabinoids, terpenes, and flavonoids work together to create an overall effect that strengthens or modifies the individual effects. Some researchers prefer the term ensemble effect, as the importance of 'minor' cannabinoids is discovered.

People choose THC-dominant strains to help manage pain, depression, anxiety, and insomnia. It is also a good choice for adult recreational use.

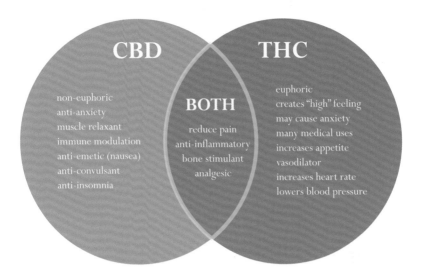

Some people feel anxious or paranoid with THC-dominant strains. They may want to choose a strain with higher levels of CBD. CBD-dominant strains have more CBD than THC. A 30:1 ratio of CBD to THC is popular. Use these strains if you need clear-headed relief.

Balanced THC/CBD strains contain equal levels of THC and CBD. These 1:1 THC/CBD formulas provide symptom relief with a mild euphoria. They may be a good choice for new consumers to try. You may develop a tolerance to the high, but the medical benefits will continue full strength.

Products with CBD and little or no THC are more widely available. Be careful, some are not as advertised and have little value. Quality CBD products will help some people; however – a little THC greatly magnifies CBD's strength. If CBD products are not working for you, you may want to try CBD with THC.

We are learning more about CBD and THC synergy all the time. Our understanding of the importance of small amounts of other cannabinoids is also growing. For example, CBG has potential health benefits aiding with skin ailments, as an antibacterial and antifungal agent.

Geek Out

The entourage effect is a synergy between cannabinoids, terpenes, and flavonoids. Some combinations magnify the effects, while others neutralize each other. Small amounts of certain cannabinoids and terpenes give cannabis superpowers over pain and ailments. Terpenes also enhance the effects. The terpene limonene, which smells like citrus, has stimulating qualities.

Mary Says: Indica, Sativa, Terpenes

I had no idea that marijuana/cannabis had different effects, different flavors, or fancy names. Frankly, when I became a consumer, I didn't care. The difference between indica and sativa was helpful. Mostly, I was interested in getting a good night's sleep, so it was indica for me. Anna is a very technical person and has been talking different cannabinoids and terpenes for a while. I told her, it was not necessary for me that beginners know this. It seemed too wonky, too much information.

I started using CBD gummies for sleep and noticed my morning stiffness in my feet went away. Huh. The stiffness in my feet comes from the cancer drugs. I noticed that when I switched to another CBD product, the stiffness came back a little. Hmm.

I have been using a THC & CBD beverage. The sleep was great, but more stiffness came back. I smoke every night now and have minor stiffness. I am sure that it is the terpenes, which vary from strain to strain. There is some difference in all the products I have tried.

This mostly creates a bigger problem. When I find some gummy or beverage or smoke I like, and there isn't detailed labeling about terpenes, how will I find that good-feeling product again? So far, I have to stick with the brands I like and hope they don't change what they are using. But until we get better analysis and labeling, it is going to be trial and error.

What Do Terpenes Do?

Terpenes do much more than give cannabis different aromas. These essential oils are also found in scented soaps, perfumes, and aromatherapies. Smells can have a powerful effect. They easily flow to the brain and trigger specific responses like alertness or sleep.

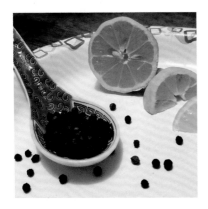

Photo: A. Sullivan

Like ingredients in a recipe, the combination of terpenes and cannabinoids produces the final result. Some terpenes help cannabinoids reach the brain and increase their potency. There is more information on specific cannabinoids and terpenes in the back of this book.

Ask about the terpenes and cannabinoids when you buy. You will find different flavors appeal to you.

Geek Out
Follow Your Nose

The terpenes in cannabis are all around us. Lavender is widely known for its calming effects because of linalool, a terpene also found in cannabis. Like spices in foods, terpenes also change cannabis effects. Smell your cannabis flower before you buy. You can learn to identify the terpenes from the smell. Here are a few regularly found in cannabis.

Citrus:	limonene	improves mood
Pine:	pinene	increases focus and memory
Mango:	myrcene	heavy sedative
Lavender:	linalool	sedative
Pepper:	caryophyllene	anti-inflammatory

Understanding Cannabis Medicine

Cannabis has been used as a medicine for centuries. Despite federal prohibition, there are many stories of people overcoming illness using cannabis medicine. However, cannabis is not a magic cure-all.

The healing benefits of cannabis were well known until the 1930s. From 1854 to 1941 cannabis was the primary medicine for over 100 separate diseases in the US Pharmacopeia. Medical textbooks from the 1920s often had a chapter dedicated to cannabis medicines.

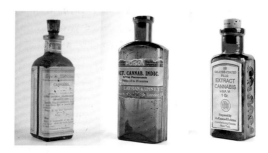

Photos courtesy of Hash Marihuana & Hemp Museum

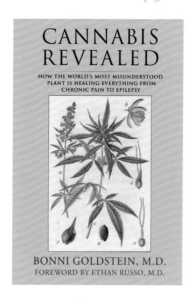

Image courtesy of Bonni Goldstein, MD Inc

Cannabis research has been limited since the 1930s. Even so, doctors frequently publish reports showing the medical properties of cannabis. There are over 30,000 studies on medicinal cannabis.

There are several good books on the medical uses of cannabis written by experienced doctors. Dr. Bonni Goldstein and her patients are featured in the new movie *Weed the People*.

Advocacy groups like NORML and Realm of Caring have online collections of cannabis research listed by diseases. This research shows that cannabinoids have many medicinal properties from anti-inflammatory to anti-depressant. Groups like NORML have been advocating for safe access to cannabis medicine for decades.

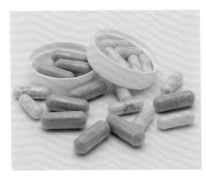

Despite prohibition, the US FDA approved two cannabis medicines. Marinol®, a synthetic THC in pill form, was approved in 1985 for nausea and vomiting related to cancer chemotherapy. In 2018, Epidiolex®, made from CBD oil, was approved to treat two rare forms of childhood epilepsy. However, the US federal government still lists cannabis as a dangerous drug.

Photo: A. Sullivan

We are still overcoming the stigma from prohibition. Some doctors are limited in what they know or can say about medicinal cannabis due to federal prohibition. You will have to decide what is right for you and your family.

> "Cannabis is remarkably safe. Although not harmless, it is surely less toxic than most of the conventional medicines it could replace if it were legally available. Despite its use by millions of people over thousands of years, cannabis has never caused an overdose death."
>
> - Dr. Lester Grinspoon, MD, Harvard University

Word To The Wise: Drug Interaction

While cannabis is non-toxic, there can be adverse drug interactions between cannabis and pharmaceuticals. You can think of cannabis like grapefruit, to be avoided with certain medications.

When you eat cannabis, like gummies or drinks, it is processed by the liver. This can change the level of other medications in your blood to inappropriately high levels. It can also interfere with the absorption of some medications, causing them to be less effective. Check with your medical provider.

Geek Out: Medicinal Properties

Research has shown **cannabinoids** to be:
Analgesic
Anti-anxiety
Anti-bacterial
Anti-cancer
Anti-convulsive
Anti-depressant
Anti-emetic (nausea)
Anti-fungal
Anti-inflammatory
Anti-insomnia
Anti-spasmodic
Appetite stimulant
Bone stimulant
Bronchodilator
Immuno-suppressive
Neuroprotective

Cannabis Tales: We Are All Made Of Star Stuff

Carl Sagan, scientist and astronomer, taught at both Harvard and Cornell. 500 million people around the world saw his TV show, **Cosmos**. Carl Sagan was a cannabis enthusiast, but had to hide it, due to his NASA security clearance. Anonymously he wrote: "The illegality of cannabis is outrageous, an impediment to full utilization of a drug which helps produce the serenity and insight, sensitivity and fellowship so desperately needed in this increasingly mad and dangerous world."

SISTERS SAY

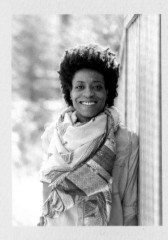

*Photo courtesy of
Trella Technologies, LLC*

Aja Atwood
Founder, Trella Technologies, LLC

What is your cannabis journey?

I was dealing with some sports injuries; I played women's tackle football. The injuries came back and I was looking for pain relief, specifically from TMJ. In 2013/14, the doctors wanted me to use prescription pain relievers, but I wanted a holistic approach. I tried ibuprofen and physical therapy, but they did not help. Then I tried cannabis; I was familiar with the plant, but was unfamiliar with its medical benefits. It worked to relieve my pain.

At the time, I was part of a technology startup doing tech around growing plants. I took a class and fell in love with the process of growing cannabis plants. I also had a full time job and was traveling a lot, managing a group of engineers from Maine to DC. I could not keep up with my plants. You have to train a plant and maintain it just about every day.

I thought, there has to be an automated system to train a plant. I researched and there was not. So I asked my friend, "Could we do that?" And he said "Hell yeah!" Now, our company, Trella Technologies, is on our 5th demo model and working on investment funding.

What is your favorite?

I like how complex the plant is, I really do. It's ironic that this plant that people are forcing into a one-size-fits-all box, is so complex; and it can't be put in a box. That speaks to me about life and freedom. It is a free plant.

What do you want people to know?

That fact that we already have a cannabinoid system in our body speaks volumes. We have receptors, ready to receive these types of molecules. It's not foreign to our body. It's a plant that assists, enhances, and enables us.

HOW TO USE CANNABIS

There is so much more to cannabis than smoking a joint. You can benefit from
the essential oils in cannabis using salves or creams, eating or drinking infused
products, or vaporizing flower or concentrates. Many find low-dose edibles
or creams are a good way to begin to experiment with cannabis.

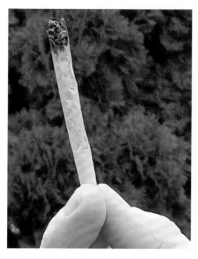

Photo: *A. Sullivan*

Did You Know?
Smoking cannabis flower is not the
same as smoking tobacco. Smoke
from cannabis does contain parti-
cles, which can irritate your throat
and lungs. However, cannabis has
not been shown to cause lung cancer
and the other diseases associated
with smoking tobacco. It is not as
physically addictive as tobacco.

Smoking cannabis flower is the most
common way to consume. Burning
the dried flower releases the essen-
tial oils and activates the THC. When you inhale the smoke, the oils can
quickly enter your blood stream. You can feel the effect of the cannabis in
a few minutes.

Because you can feel the effects right away, you can easily control how much
you are getting. If you want more, take another toke, puff, or hit. If you had
enough, you can pass.

The cannabis flower is the most basic form of cannabis. All other products
are made from flower. Usually, at the dispensary, there will be more varieties
of flower than edibles or tinctures to choose from. It may be easier to find
the varieties that are right for you.

Processing flower changes the essentials oils and may add things you don't
want. Some extraction methods change the mix of essential oils in the raw
flower and may leave residuals. Some edibles are high in sugar. Ask questions
when you buy.

Did You Know?

You can enjoy cannabis by soaking in it. Companies combine cannabis and essential oils in bath salts. Soaking in a medicated bath provides deep relaxation and relief from aches and pains. Some are specifically designed to help women find relief from menstrual cramping.

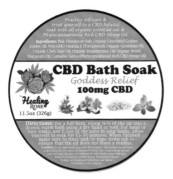 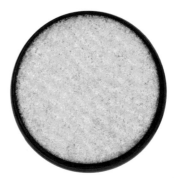

Photos courtesy of The Healing Rose

Buzz Words

Flower: The bud of the cannabis plant, typically smoked or vaporized.

Edible: A food or drink infused with cannabis oils.

Concentrate: Oils extracted from cannabis flower, typically smoked or vaporized.

Tincture: Typically an alcohol extraction, usually put in your mouth to absorb.

Topical: A cream or salve used on your skin.

Look for cannabis tested at an independent lab. Ask about the test results. Sample cannabis test results are included in the Appendix. Often they show the percent of the primary cannabinoids (THC, CBD, CBG) and terpenes. It is also important to check for residual pesticides and solvents.

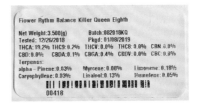

Photo: A. Sullivan

Cannabis produces different durations and effects depending on whether it is smoked or eaten. When you smoke, cannabis enters your blood stream immediately through your lungs. You feel the effect right away. An edible is processed in the stomach and liver. The effects are delayed. Cannabis absorbed in your mouth is not processed by the digestive system. Drops under the tongue or lozenges are quickly absorbed into your blood stream via the mucous membranes under your tongue.

Type	Method	Effects	Duration	Benefits
Flower	Inhale	3 - 5 minutes	½ - 2 hours	Easy to control
Edible	Ingest	30 - 120 minutes	3+ hours	No inhalation, longer lasting
Concentrate	Inhale	3 - 5 minutes	½ - 2 hours	Stronger effect
Tincture	Under tongue	15 - 60 minutes	1 - 4 hours	No inhalation, longer lasting
Topical	Apply to skin	20 - 120 minutes	1 - 4 hours	Targeted relief, no high
Transdermal	Apply patch to skin	15 - 30 minutes	6 - 8 hours	Strong long lasting

How do the cannabinoids get to where they are going? How fast and how directly do they get into your blood stream? Cannabinoids enter the blood stream faster through mucous membranes than through your skin. Understanding modes of consumption will help you choose what to use. You may want different products at different times of the day.

Topicals are becoming popular. A cream or salve will have a localized effect. Apply directly to affected areas. Creams may relieve rashes in addition to calming aching muscles.

Word to the Wise

Cannabis is a euphoric, which could trigger dependence. Although some people who consume cannabis may become dependent, it is at a much lower rate than alcohol, tobacco, or opioids.

Alcohol, tobacco, and opioids cause physical addition, while marijuana dependence is primarily psychological. Cannabis withdrawal may include headaches and grouchiness, but typically not vomiting and muscle spasms.

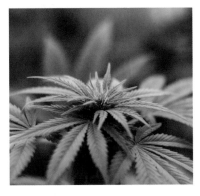

Image courtesy of Bask Inc

More medicinal ways of consuming cannabis include the following: drops from a calibrated syringe placed under your tongue, transdermal patches, and suppositories. Medicinal doses can be much stronger than the 'typical' 5 or 10 mg serving set by state regulatory agencies.

Cannabis is personalized medicine. Some people are more sensitive to THC. Your ECS, cannabis uptake, and reactions are different depending on genetics, hormones, diet, and exercise. Various strains of cannabis will have different effects. How you consume also plays a factor. Unlike a rigid pill prescription, you need to experiment with cannabis to see what works for you.

Think about what you want from cannabis. Medicating to relieve pain or anxiety is different than enjoying an evening with friends. A soak or a cream will ease aching muscles, while a candy or pill might be just right at bedtime.

Mary Says: Cannabis As Part Of Cancer Treatment

The side effects of the anticancer drugs, the cocktail, can be overwhelming. Every ache and pain could be side effects, cancer, or conditions caused by a side effect. For example, dizziness could be caused by low blood sugar from lack of food, lack of appetite, or ongoing nausea.

I have trouble sleeping for many reasons. I feel that good sleep is so important for health. I started with CBD gummies from a local shop. I mostly used the same brand. I was not worried about sugar as I was only having one 10 mg gummy each night. One of my cancer drug side effects is hyper substance sensitivity. I would eat the gummies and be asleep in 15 minutes, sleeping deeply thru the night.

When I decided I no longer needed morphine, I tried quitting cold turkey. I had little effects from withdrawal but they included a skin-crawling sensation. One CBD gummy took away that skin-crawling feeling. I took more CBD during that time, but it was very worth the liberation from morphine.

Smoking Flower: Joints

Rolling a cannabis cigarette or joint is the most common way to consume cannabis. That may change as legalization spreads and new products become available. All you need are papers, a lighter, and cannabis. Doobies, bones, cones, and pre-rolls are all different names for the simple joint.

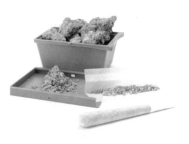

Photo courtesy of Sana Packaging

Rolling papers come in a variety of sizes and quality. Some people prefer unbleached papers. You can typically buy rolling papers where tobacco is sold. It is handy to roll over a tray, as it can be messy.

Each paper has a crease. One side has gum like an envelope. Simply break or grind the cannabis into small pieces and put it in the crease. Roll the paper tightly around the flower, lick the gum, and seal. It is a balance to make it tight enough to stay together and loose enough to get a good draw after you light it.

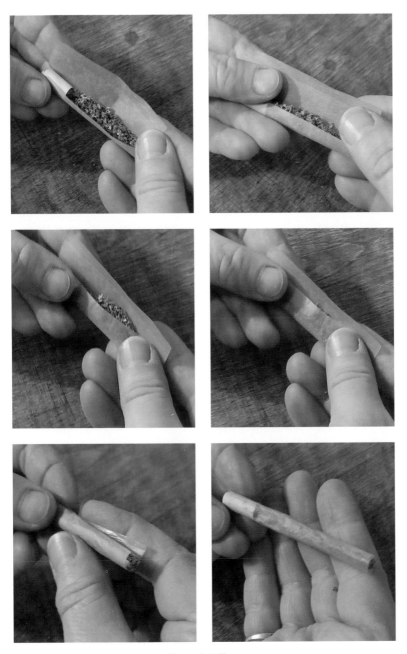

Photos: A. Sullivan

Over the years, people have developed helpful gadgets. Grinders and rolling machines may make rolling joints easier.

> **Must Haves!**
>
> It is a good idea to have a mat or tray to contain the herb when grinding, rolling a joint, or filling a pipe. Herb on the floor is a lost cause. A magazine is often handy.

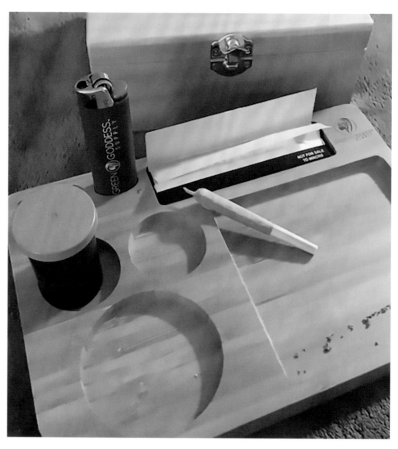

Photo courtesy of Green Goddess Supply

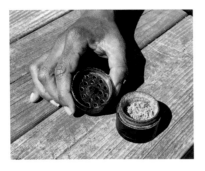

Photo courtesy of Trella Technologies, LLC

The joint will burn more evenly if the cannabis is in uniformly small pieces.

Modern flower is dense with terpenes and tends to be sticky. You grind the herb or crush the bud with your fingers to form small chunks. A grinder helps break the buds and give you a more even joint.

The end of a joint, or roach, can be difficult to smoke. Some use a roach clip to hold the small butt. Some people like to add a filter, tip, or crutch to the end of the joint to make it easier to hold.

Did You Know?

A spliff is a joint that is part cannabis and part tobacco. Tobacco can be rolled with flower, hash, or oil. In Amsterdam, it is common to see a jar of tobacco and rolling papers on the counters of the "coffee shop."

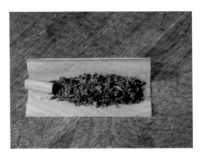

Photo: A. Sullivan

A glass crutch is a small glass tube and can be reused. However, most just roll up a piece of stiff paper instead of using a crutch. The tip is rolled into one

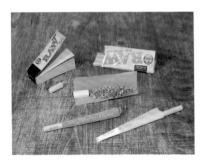

Photo: A. Sullivan

end of the joint, like a filter in a tobacco cigarette. It makes it easier to pass and smoke the end of the joint.

Now you can buy empty paper cones or blunt wraps, ready to load with cannabis. Loading the cone can be tricky. You can buy gadgets to help load the cone. Most cones come with a stick to pack the joint.

Did You Know?

Unfortunately, some cannabis is sold with lots of plastic packaging. Choose wisely. Some companies make childproof sustainable packaging for cannabis using 100% plant-based hemp or 100% reclaimed ocean plastic.

Must Haves!

Single joints, or "doobies" may be sold in a capped plastic tube. A doob tube keeps your joint from being damaged. It is a good idea to keep one around to keep your doobies safe in your pocket or bag.

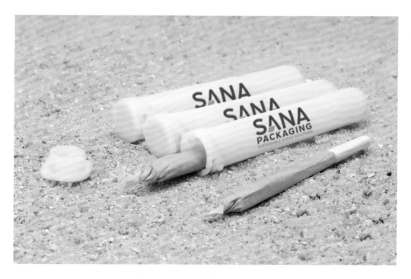

Photo courtesy of Sana Packaging

Buzz Words

Joint: Ground cannabis rolled in a paper cigarette. Can also have a glass or paper tip called a crutch or filter.

Spliff: A joint with both tobacco and cannabis, either flower or hash.

Blunt: Cannabis joint rolled into a cigar wrapper.

Pre-roll: A joint that has been commercially filled and rolled.

Must Haves!

Cannabis can involve many parts and pieces: herb, lighters, pipes, grinder, and more. It is best to have a little bag or pouch to keep everything together. Some state laws require you to lock up your stash in your home. Most people have a stash bag or two to keep everything together.

Some people use a rolling machine to roll even joints. They are available where pipes and bongs are sold. A rolling machine is fairly easy to use.

I like rolling my own joints and sometimes use a tip. Filling a paper cone didn't seem worth the effort. Dispensaries sell pre-rolls if I wanted one. Everyone has their own style. There are many variations.

Friends Say:

You can dilute smoke to get a milder hit. Take a puff into your mouth. As you hold the smoke in your mouth, inhale plain air into your lungs. This will carry the smoke into your lungs and dilute it, giving you a milder puff.

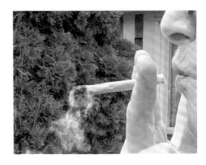

Photo: A. Sullivan

You smoke a joint like you would a cigarette. Put the filter end in your mouth and light the other end while inhaling. At first, only take a small puff or hit. Coughing a big cloud of smoke is common if you take a big hit. Joints are commonly shared. One or two puffs may be enough, save the rest for later.

Take a 2-second puff. See how you feel in 5-10 minutes. If you want, take a second puff. Wait another 5-10 minutes and see if you want another. This way you can easily tell how that strain of cannabis affects you. And you can control how much you consume.

SISTERS SAY

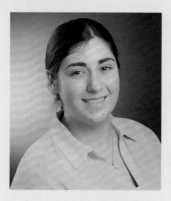

Photo courtesy of Sarah Gibbs

Sarah Gibbs
Co-Founder, Healing Tree Edibles

What is your cannabis journey?

I've been smoking since I was 15 or 16. Working as a chef, I developed shoulder and lower back pain. Topicals and smoking have helped to ease the tightness and what feels like pinching in my shoulder.

What has really motivated me to step further into the medical side of the industry has been my dad. He has severe anxiety, depression, PTSD, restless leg syndrome, and a rare disease called Wegener's Granulomatosis (he lost one of his kidneys to it in 2015).

His anxiety had gotten so bad, he was trying electroshock therapy and had lost about 50 lbs. He was on 250 mg of the anti-psychotic drug Seroquel 4 times a day.

I finally got him to start using some hemp-based CBD oil and it has helped drastically. He now only takes 75 mg of Seroquel once at night. He's been up doing things around the house and going outside again, singing and cracking jokes. Before, my mom could hardly go to the grocery store without him having a panic attack.

What is your favorite?

One of my favorite things about cannabis is that it is so versatile. It's medicine, clothing, construction materials, etc. I also love the social aspect of passing a bowl around and having a good laugh with friends and even strangers. Nothing brings people together like sharing some bud.

What is one thing you want people to know?

I want people to know there's nothing to be afraid of, but you have to know yourself and your limits. You can't just jump right in. It can be incredibly beneficial, but only when used the right ways.

Pipes

Cannabis flower can also be smoked in a pipe often called a bowl. Sharing a bowl with friends is fun. It can be a nice enhancement to many social activities from video games to hiking to painting or being creative.

Good to Know

Don't bogart the bowl. Good pipe-passing etiquette is you take a puff or two and then pass the bowl. Sometimes people will get talking or just stoned and forget to pass the bowl. Be considerate and puff, puff, pass.

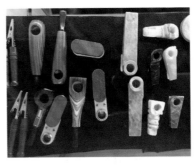

Photo: Anna Meade

Pipes or bowls come in many shapes and sizes. They can be made of wood, glass, stone, metal or plastic. I enjoy looking at all of the creative expressions and innovations when browsing in my smoke shop. I like to hold a pipe before I buy it, although you can order them online.

Buzz Words

Pipe (bowl): A device to smoke hash or flower using a flame to light the herb.

Hooka: A device to smoke that has several mouthpieces.

Bong: A water pipe; the water cools and can flavor the smoke before it is inhaled.

One-Hitter (chillum): A small pipe that holds one hit or puff.

Vaporizer: A device that heats the herb until the oils turn to steam and can be inhaled.

Hookas typically sit on a table and have several mouthpieces so a few people can use it at the same time. Pipes are smaller and passed among friends. Some pipes have a chamber to cool the smoke. Bongs cool the smoke through water or ice. The water filters some tar and ash from the smoke.

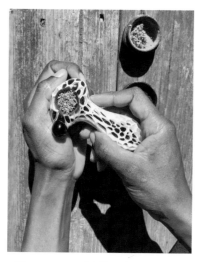

Photo courtesy of Trella Technologies, LLC

Loading a pipe is fairly straightforward. Break the cannabis into small pieces with your hands or a grinder. Place them into the bowl of the pipe. Pack it a little so it burns smoothly. You inhale from the mouthpiece while lighting the herb in the bowl.

Some pipes and bongs have a small hole on the side called a carburetor or carb. You place your finger over the hole upon initial draw, filling the pipe with smoke. When you are almost done, you lift your finger and continue drawing. This allows clean air in, and clears the chamber.

Friends Say

Remember, when you are lighting a bowl you are also inhaling the exhaust from the lighter. Many choose butane gas over fluid lighters because they burn cleaner. Some purists use a hemp wick dipped in bees wax, lit by a candle.

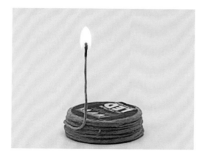

Photo: A. Sullivan

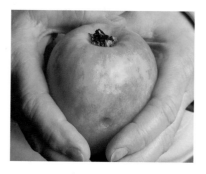

Photo: A. Sullivan

Did You Know?

You can make a pipe out of anything! Cannabis paraphernalia was difficult to get for many years. People got very creative making pipes from apples, soda cans, beakers, fruit, or anything around home or campus.

Bongs

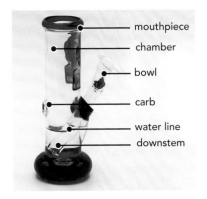

mouthpiece
chamber
bowl
carb
water line
downstem

Photo: A. Sullivan

A bong is a water pipe. They are made of glass, plastic, metal, or a combination. Bongs are clear, colored, or decorated with everything from skulls to sports team emblems. With so many shapes and sizes, shopping can be fun.

The base of the bong is filled with water or ice. Flavoring can be added. The water level should be above the bottom of the downstem and below the carb hole.

Fill the bowl with cannabis. Unlike a pipe, often a bong bowl will not have a screen. Use pieces that are larger than the hole. Some bongs only hold one puff or hit.

If it has one, place your finger over the carb. Hold the lighter by the bowl and inhale through the mouthpiece, lighting the herb. The smoke will be drawn through the water and into the chamber.

Once you fill the chamber with smoke, move your finger off the carb and inhale. This way you inhale the smoke from the chamber into your lungs. For some bongs, you lift the bowl to clear the chamber. On some glass bongs you lift the whole downstem, called a slide.

Some people stop and exhale to clear their lungs after filling the chamber. This allows a larger hit. It is poor form to leave smoke in the bong as you pass it.

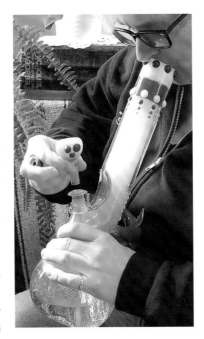

Photo: A. Sullivan

37

Vaporizers

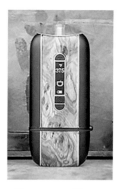

Relatively new on the scene are dry flower vaporizers or furnaces. These machines heat the flower until the essential oils turn into steam and can be inhaled. However, the cannabis leaves are not burned. This provides a cleaner smoke without the ash from burning leaves or paper.

The various essential oils in cannabis vaporize at different temperatures. Charts on the following page and in the Appendix show the different vaporization temperatures. Some models have adjustable settings.

Photo courtesy of Davinci

Ask questions before you buy so you understand all the features.

Vaporizers come in several sizes, both hand held and table models. Some can be pricey. The high-end models have Bluetooth and can be programmed with your phone. Some have a compartment to store a refill. Vaporizers are electronic and have to be charged periodically.

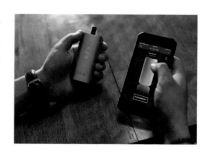

Photo courtesy of Davinci

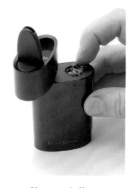

Follow the directions as machines differ slightly for packing and heating the bowl. Grind the flower into fine pieces. Some use a coffee grinder. Pack the bowl and turn it on. You have to wait while the cannabis is heated. A green light typically means it is ready to smoke.

Some table models have a removable chamber. Once it fills with vapor, you can remove it and inhale. Others have a mouthpiece. I enjoy the clean smoke, just the good stuff and no ash.

Photo: A. Sullivan

WHAT'S YOUR PATH?

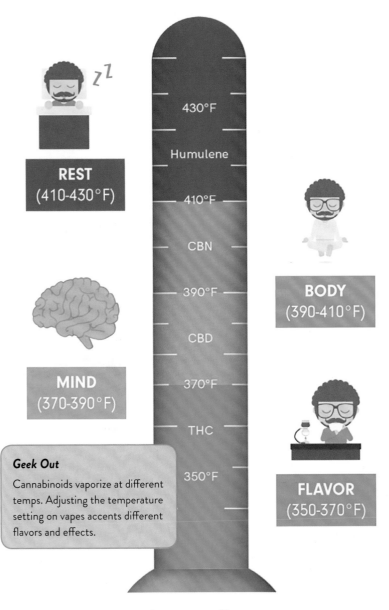

REST
(410-430°F)

MIND
(370-390°F)

430°F

Humulene

410°F

CBN

390°F

CBD

370°F

THC

350°F

BODY
(390-410°F)

FLAVOR
(350-370°F)

Geek Out

Cannabinoids vaporize at different temps. Adjusting the temperature setting on vapes accents different flavors and effects.

Image courtesy of Davinci

Cleaning

Periodically you need to clean your pipes and bongs. Clean the ash out of the bowl after all the cannabis is burned before refilling it. Usually tapping it in the ashtray is enough. Change the bong water regularly. Your smoke will taste better and your friends will thank you.

Bongs and pipes get coated with a sticky tar called resin. The tar and ash can clog the stem and screen. If it is hard to draw, it is time to clean!

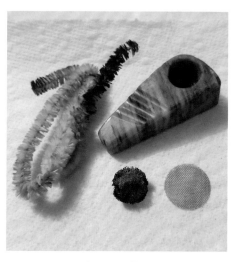

Clean the bowl. Remove the screen. Scrape the ash and tar off the screen. Replace it if necessary. Screens are inexpensive; I try to always have an extra. Scrape the tar and ash from the inside of the bowl. Be careful not to chip it.

Photo: A. Sullivan

Cleaning the inside of your pipe can be challenging. Specialty cleaners can work wonders. You can also use rubbing alcohol or hot water to dissolve the tar inside the pipe.

> **Word to the Wise**
>
> Cannabis tar is sticky and stinky. Be careful it doesn't get all over when you are cleaning. Bong water can also be nasty, especially if spilled on the carpet.

Use pipe cleaners or cotton swabs to wipe the inside. You can straighten a paper clip to clear the stem. Personally, I use rubbing alcohol and pipe cleaners.(Pipe cleaners are also fun for craft projects.)

If you cover the work area with paper towels or newspapers, the mess is easier to clean up.

To clean with alcohol, put isopropyl alcohol and your pipe into a baggie. Seal it and shake it, so the mixture fills the pipe. Let it sit for 30 minutes.

Any residue comes off with pipe cleaners. I like to rinse my pipe with alcohol again after using pipe cleaners. Be sure to rinse your pipe well with water before using it again.

Another method is to simmer it in hot water for 30 minutes. For the simmering method, put the bowl in a pot with cold water. Turn on the

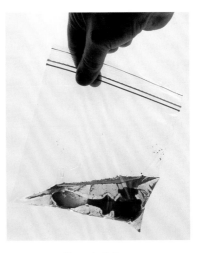

Photo: A. Sullivan

heat so it gradually starts to simmer. The hot water will dissolve the tar. Use an old pan — you may not want to use it for cooking afterwards.

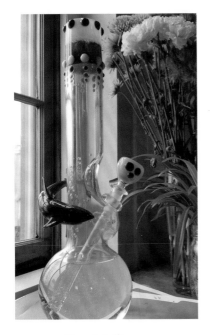

Photo: A. Sullivan

Word to the Wise
Glass pipes and bongs are fragile. Be careful when cleaning glass, you can easily crack, chip, or break it.

Edibles

The essential oils in cannabis can be removed from the plant and used to make food. Cannabis-infused foods are called edibles. Pot brownies are legendary, but the new legal market includes everything from cookies to drinks to BBQ sauce and rubs.

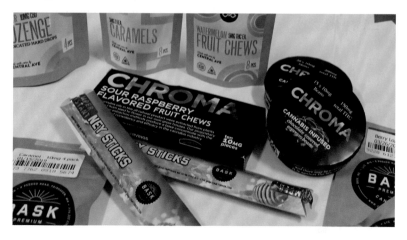

Photo: Anna Meade

The essential oils, cannabinoids, terpenes, and flavonoids dissolve in fats or alcohol. They can be easily infused into butter or oils and used to make any foods that include butter or oil. The cannabis must be heated before using it to infuse oils. Heating cannabis is called decarboxylation; it changes or activates the THC so it has a euphoric effect.

Word to the Wise

Not Too Much

The most common mistake is eating too much edibles. People have a little bit, feel nothing, and eat more. And then they feel sick. Edibles take from 30 to 120 minutes to take effect.

Start low, go slow.

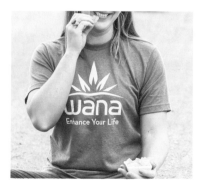

Photo courtesy of Wana Brands

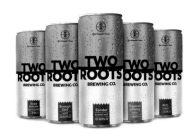

Photo courtesy of Two Roots

New products are launched daily. Cookies, brownies, and candies are popular and available in most dispensaries. Cannabis chefs are infusing a variety of foods for those who want to go beyond sweets. Cannabis drinks are becoming very popular. Several types of sodas are available as well as non-alcoholic beers.

Before you eat an edible, determine how much cannabis is in it. Find out the suggested serving and dosage. Start low and go slow.

Products sold in dispensaries are typically labeled with the amount of THC in each serving and per container. A serving size of THC or CBD is 5 or 10 mg. If you are new, start with one serving or less. Some feel high with 1 mg of THC. Everyone is different.

A chocolate bar may have 10 pieces. Each piece is a 10 mg serving. A whole chocolate bar may have 100 mg; the amount should be marked on the label. Eating the entire bar may make you feel sick. If you are not sure of the dosage in a product, ask questions before you buy.

States may limit the amount of THC that one package can contain. This may differ for medicinal use items.

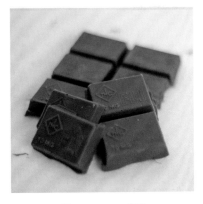

Photo courtesy of Fli

Similar to alcohol, the effects you experience may vary depending on whether your stomach is full or empty, if consumed with alcohol or fats, and your personal tolerance level.

It can be difficult to know the strength of homemade edibles. Ask how much cannabis flower was used for each batch. You can use the sample formula on page 45 to estimate the potency of homemade brownies.

When you eat cannabis-infused foods, they are digested and enter your blood stream. Digestion changes the cannabinoids to be much stronger. Cannabis will have a noticeable effect once it is in your blood stream. This may take 30 minutes or up to an hour for the full effect.

The high you get from edibles may differ from smoking. Each consumption method affects you differently.

Typically, the effects last longer than when you smoke cannabis. Edibles may get you high for up to 4 hours. This is great for a day at the beach or evening. Be careful and plan for how long the effects might last.

Some people panic when they consume too much. The good news is that it will wear off in a few hours. There are no lasting side effects from getting way too high. There are no known deaths from an overdose of cannabis. Take a cool bath or get outside and walk. Fresh air can help reduce paranoia.

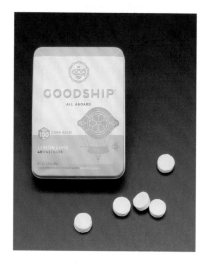

Photo: A. Sullivan

Cannabis Tales:

Pot Brownies

Many credit Alice B. Toklas with inventing pot brownies. Toklas was Gertrude Stein's partner. Their regular salons in Paris attracted writers and artists like Picasso, Ernest Hemingway, Thornton Wilder, and Matisse.

In 1954, Toklas published a cookbook. The Hashish Fudge recipe with spices, nuts, fruit, and cannabis caused a stir. Toklas wrote that the fudge is easy to whip up on a rainy day and can liven up any gathering. The book and the fudge were quite popular.

"Euphoria and brilliant storms of laughter; estatic reveries and extensions of one's personality on several simultaneous planes are to be complacently expected."

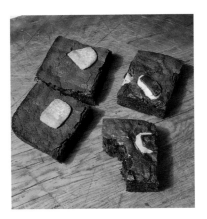

Photo: A. Sullivan

Example For Dosing Homemade Infused Brownies

First decarboxylate your cannabis by baking it for ~30 mins at 220 ° F, to activate the THC.

Infuse **1 gram of flower per stick of butter**. There are 1,000 mg in a gram. Average THC is 10%. 10% of 1,000 is 100 mg. One stick of butter will have 100 mg.

Each stick has 8 Tbs. Divide 100 mg by 8 Tbs = **12.5 mg of THC per Tbs of butter.**

Brownies take 5 Tbs of butter.

5 Tbs x 12.5 mg/Tbs = 62.5 mg/ mix.

Cut brownies into 9 pieces. Each piece of brownie will have 7 mg of THC.

Friends Say

When you make cannabis brownies, make another batch of brownies without cannabis. People can enjoy an additional brownie and not consume too much cannabis.

45

SISTERS SAY

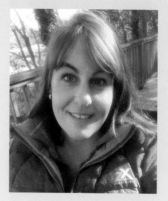

Photo courtesy of Mikki Bennett

Mikki Bennett
Founder of Healing Tree Edibles

What is your cannabis journey?

I have always been a cook, so when I got injured and broke my ankle, the guy I worked for brought me a bunch of chocolates. Turns out they were infused with THC and helped me manage my pain without opiates.

I took one chocolate every six hours in place of a Percocet even though I had a 6-inch plate with seven screws in my ankle and I was bedridden for six months. Cannabis carried me through it.

I come from a long line of short stocky Italians who are diabetics. I wanted to create something that provided medicine without all the sugar and fat that diabetics can't have. That's when I created infused granola and granola bars.

That's what did it for me. Once I created that, I figured it was a healing thing. So it was a healthy way to heal; a healthy way to treat your pain, your aches, your ailments. Prior to this injury, I had only smoked cannabis on occasion to battle depression and keep me off of antidepressants.

Now Healing Tree Edibles is creating healthy options for others. Many people don't want to smoke, but they still need natural medicine. People don't have to have junk food or cookies with high sugar and high fat. We are giving them an alternative, using organic ingredients and gluten-free ingredients.

What is your favorite?

I like food when you can taste the food, not medicine. So we tend to do flavorful and savory foods like our Chex Mix. That's one of my favorites; just a couple pieces and you are good for several hours. Our Crab Rangoons are a close second.

What do you want to tell people?

I feel the most important thing that anyone could ever understand when it comes to edibles is how to properly dose yourself. Too many people think that they have a much higher tolerance than they actually do. The other problem is people don't take into account whether or not their stomach is empty or the lag time before you feel the effects. In most cases, it can be close to two hours. People want instant gratification and you don't get that by eating edibles.

Vaping Cartridges

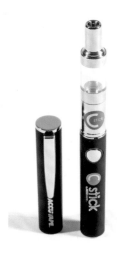

Extracting the oils from the cannabis flower creates a high potency concentrate. Similar to nicotine cartridges used with electronic cigarettes, cannabis oils are loaded into cartridges or carts. A pen battery is used to heat the oil till it vaporizes. You inhale through the mouthpiece. It can be an easy and discreet way to consume cannabis.

There are a various types of batteries and cartridges on the market. Some are refillable. Standard 1 gram and 0.5 gram disposable carts with a rechargeable battery base are becoming popular. Check to see if the carts you buy work with your battery base.

Photo courtesy of AccuVape

The battery base must be charged. Many pens come with a USB charger base. Others plug into the wall.

The cart is screwed onto the battery base. Some carts have protective caps for the base and mouthpiece. I like to store my carts in their case with the protective caps on.

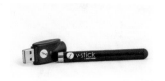

Photo courtesy of AccuVape

Photo courtesy of AccuVape

The battery heats the oil until it vaporizes, like water turns into steam. It won't burn as you inhale. You'll taste the flavor profile of the cannabis oil. You are not inhaling ash like smoking. There is little residual smell, which makes it a discreet way to consume.

Some are easy to use — just puff on them until you see the vapor. A button activates others. Regulating the temperature enhances cannabinoid and flavor profiles. Ask how to use one before buying it.

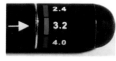

Photo courtesy of AccuVape

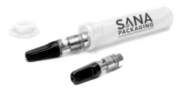

Photo courtesy of Sana Packaging

Several methods are used to extract oil from cannabis. Butane, CO_2, alcohol, and heat press are common. Certain methods keep the cannabinoids but not the terpenes. Some manufacturers add terpenes, flavors, or thinners into the oil to flavor or thin it. Some additives, like propylene glycol, are not safe to heat and inhale. Full spectrum oils contain all of the oils from the plant.

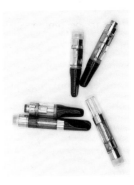

Photo: A. Sullivan

Choose vape carts that are lab tested for purity and that contain cannabis grown without pesticides.

For your first try, take a small puff. A two second draw is good. Wait till you feel an effect. One, maybe two puffs are enough for people who do not smoke regularly.

Other concentrates are produced by different extraction methods. Concentrates are very strong and not recommended for new users.

Topicals

You can absorb cannabis through your skin. It will not get you high, but it may provide relief for aching muscles and joints. Cannabis-infused creams are called topicals and come in many varieties.

Cannabis-infused coconut oil is a common base for creams and salves. Shea butter, jojoba, eucalyptus, and other healing oils are often included in creams or lotions. Salves are wax based and may include menthol to stimulate blood flow to the area. Both are useful to get targeted relief to the skin or muscles.

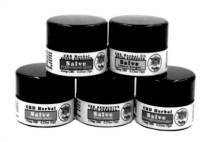

Photo courtesy of The Healing Rose

Creams offer localized pain and muscle relief. Cannabis cream can be used to alleviate eczema, psoriasis, and skin irritations. Some formulations are good for minor burns or dry itchy skin. Creams can also be rubbed into achy muscles. Massage therapists offer treatments with infused massage oils.

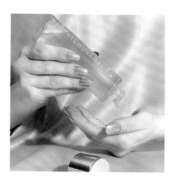 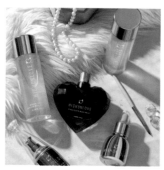

Photos courtesy of Love and Beauty Products

Infused bath bombs are becoming very popular. Some combine aromatherapy for a relaxing or invigorating bath. Epsom salts enhance the healing properties of cannabis. An infused bath is a great way to unwind after work or heal the body after a hard workout. Many women enjoy infused sensual products.

Medicinals

Over 2 million people in the US are using medical marijuana through state programs. California legalized medical marijuana in 1996 and has been joined by 32 states. The laws are changing regularly; however, it is still illegal in some states and at the federal level.

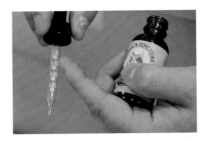

Photo: Anna Meade

Different products have been developed to supply medical marijuana. There are ways to get lasting effects when inhalation is not appropriate. Pills, tablets, and lozenges are familiar ways to consume medicine. Cannabis tinctures taken by mouth or in food are common.

Droppers deliver measured amounts of tinctures or oils, which adds more accuracy to dosing. Accurate dosing is important in medical uses and can be challenging.

Transdermal patches on the skin allow cannabinoids to reach your blood stream. Suppositories get cannabis into your blood stream without being processed by the digestive system. This provides discreet long-lasting relief.

Flower, edibles, tinctures, and concentrates are also available for medical uses. Micro-dosing can manage minor symptoms; more serious medical uses may require higher doses. Consult a medical professional. Start low and see if cannabis is right for you.

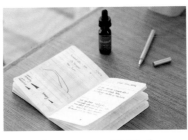

Image courtesy of Goldleaf

A cannabis consumption journal can help you determine what products and dosing are right for you. Many dispensaries provide a simple journal. A sample is included in the Appendix. Apps can also help you track your purchases and how they make you feel.

51

SISTERS SAY

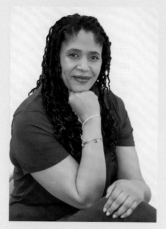

Photo courtesy of Golden Piff

Golden Piff
Urban Cannabis
GrowOp Association

What is your cannabis journey?

Marijuana as a viable medical option wasn't something that crossed this mom's mind — until 2001 when my child went down to 70 lbs. and we discovered that she had cancerous polyps: cannabis became an option. Without definitive answers on the effect marijuana treatments would have on her, I knew I had to be willing to save my child's life; risk be damned.

I followed the recommendations of her oncologist and began treating her in order to stimulate her appetite. Her progress is what has pushed me to continually understand the benefits of marijuana and further enter the newly regulated industry — to ensure I am in a position to show others the positive benefits of cannabis.

A few years after my daughter's severe health complications, I was injured in such a way as to cause a traumatic brain injury. I was told I would not be able to talk, I would not be able to walk, and that my life would be forever changed - I turned to cannabis in my time of need. Marijuana saved my life.

Traditional medication was not the answer for me; I had children I was fighting to be present for and being in a medically induced psychosis was going to alter our family's quality of life. I have been prescription free for 10 years and I proudly consume cannabis, maintain a full time job, and those children have blessed me with the most beautiful grandchildren; I get to actively be a part of their lives.

My Great Grandmother was a black female entrepreneur and community leader during a time when she was told she couldn't be — breaking boundaries is in my blood. I plan to carry on her legacy as I enter the Massachusetts Recreational Cannabis Industry by forming the first black owned and operated cannabis cooperative in Massachusetts. Together we will continue her 120-year legacy of cultivating community on our family's land.

Though I will begin by establishing the cooperative, I believe my mission is much larger and I look forward to working across Massachusetts and states far beyond, on marijuana conviction expungement and equitable access for disproportionately harmed communities to enter legal marijuana markets.

What is your favorite?

My favorite part of being a part of the cannabis industry is having the opportunity to share the positive benefits of marijuana with those who might not have an opportunity to be exposed to the layers of benefits of the plant in its entirety. From the positive effects on the cannabinoid system to bringing real change to disproportionately harmed communities, I love to motivate people to learn more about marijuana.

What do you want people to know?

If I want people to know anything, it's that they have an incredible power; and they have the ability to use that power to learn about the propaganda that has been spoon fed to us about marijuana. If we are willing to learn about weed, we will break the stigma and begin to collectively benefit from cannabis.

Cannabis Tales: Killing Cancer with Cannabis

Dr. Dedi Meiri of Israel is a world-renowned scientist on the effects of cannabis on cancer cells. His team isolates the different compounds to see what is effective. His research shows that certain combinations of cannabinoids and terpenes will slow cancer cell growth and motility and kill certain cancer cells in a petri dish. It's a long way from human treatments.

There is much promise; but there are 100 different types of cancer and a million combinations of cannabinoids. Research is ongoing.

Cannabis is, however, generally accepted as an effective treatment for some of the side effects of chemotherapy: reducing nausea, stimulating appetite, and managing pain. Some studies suggest that cannabinoids improve the efficacy of radiation therapy.

Mary Says: Cannabis cures cancer?

This is so offensive to many cancer patients. The inference is that cannabis is a miracle ignored. Only people who have not been diagnosed with cancer think that there are secret untried cancer treatments. Every cancer patient gets messages from friends about those cures. I have a terminal disease but people, even strangers, tell me that I missed this or that miracle. The idea that I am not doing everything I can to get well is deeply hurtful, ignorant, and moves me to anger.

Cancer is a general term: there are nine subtypes of breast cancer. Is it hard to believe that one drug or herb will cure cancers which are so different? Some cancers are very specific and act the same in everyone. Breast cancer, in addition to sub-types, has many different genetic markers to mix and match with the sub-types. Some are aggressive and some are slow moving; some hurt and some do not.

Cannabis has a huge place in cancer treatment, but there are very few "cures."

HOW TO GET YOUR MEDICAL MARIJUANA CARD

Medical marijuana programs are run by state governments and differ slightly. Check your local laws. Some states limit medical marijuana to specific illnesses, while others are very broad.

Most have a website which explains the process. Typically, there are two steps: 1) Get a doctor's recommendation. 2) Apply online to the state to get a medical marijuana card.

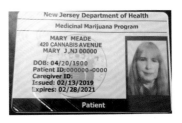

Image courtesy of M. Meade

Some doctors and nurses specialize in cannabis medicine. Finding a doctor to make a recommendation is fairly easy. The state or private websites will list doctors who recommend medical marijuana.

Medical marijuana has been recommended for over 250 different medical conditions. Be sure to consult a doctor or nurse to treat complex illnesses.

Some people already have a medical care team and just need an official recommendation. You may be able to get a recommendation without an office visit. You may need to provide your medical records.

Good to know

1. The doctor's visit may cost $100-$250 dollars and is generally not covered by insurance.

2. Medical cannabis is generally not covered by insurance.

3. Medical cards may need to be renewed every year.

4. You may have to prove residency.

5. Some programs offer a financial hardship waiver of the fees.

6. A few states honor other states' medical marijuana cards, which is useful when you travel.

> **Buzz Words**
>
> **Qualifying Condition**: Many states list specific medical conditions for which marijuana may be recommended.
>
> **Medical Marijuana**: Any cannabis product or flower used for medicinal purposes.
>
> **Doctor's Recommendation**: A written statement by a qualified medical professional (doctor or nurse) stating that marijuana could help the patient.
>
> **Medical Marijuana Card**: A state-issued photo ID used to allow access to medical marijuana dispensaries in certain states.

Once you have your doctor's recommendation, you will need to complete the state application online. Usually there is a fee. Most require proof of residency. Some doctors will complete the online application with you.

Once you have a card, you may purchase any type and quantity of cannabis products at a dispensary. There are legal limits for individual purchases. Called reciprocity, many states will honor other states' medical marijuana cards.

Many patients use cannabis instead of certain prescription drugs and for drug dependence withdrawal. Working with a licensed professional is recommended. Some states will allow you to exchange an opioid prescription for cannabis medicine.

> **Did You Know?**
>
> **Plants vs Pharma**: Pharmaceutical companies isolate and test one or two compounds to determine dosing and expected effects. Cannabis medicines use many if not all of the compounds in the plant. Cannabis medicine is more personal than "Take three pills every four hours." You may need to experiment to know what works for you. You may need to adjust your consumption to manage symptoms.

Did You Know?

THE MOST COMMON QUALIFYING CONDITIONS ARE:

Arthritis

Cancer

Chronic Pain

Crohn's Disease

Epilepsy

Fibromyalgia

Glaucoma

HIV/AIDS

Multiple Sclerosis (MS)

Nausea

PTSD

ADDITIONAL QUALIFYING CONDITIONS INCLUDE:

Acid Reflux

Acne

Alcoholism

Alzheimer's Disease

Anorexia

Anxiety Disorder

Asthma

ADD & ADHD

Autoimmune Disease

Back Pain

Bipolar Disorder

Broken Bones

Carpal Tunnel Syndrome

Chemotherapy

Chronic Fatigue Syndrome

Concussions

Constipation

Dementia

Depression

Diabetes

Digestive Disorders

Eczema

Headaches

High Blood Pressure

Impotence

Inflammation

Inflammatory Bowel Disease

Insomnia

Lyme Disease

Menstrual Cramps

Mood Disorders

Motion Sickness

Muscle Spasms

Neuropathy

Nicotine or Opiate Dependence

Parkinson's Disease

Schizophrenia

Seizures

Skin Disease

Sleep Disorders

Stress

Stroke

Thyroid Disorders

Traumatic Brain Injury

Tremors

Tumors

Ulcers

Vomiting

Writer's Cramp

SHOPPING AT A DISPENSARY

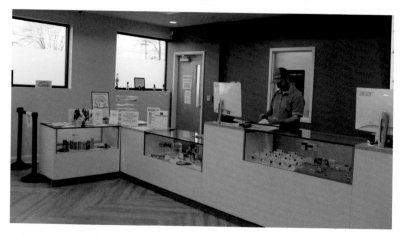

Photo: Anna Meade

Some dispensaries have the sleek stylings of high-end retail tech stores. Products are displayed in enclosed cabinets with plenty of browsing room. Sales staff guide you through the facility.

Dispensaries have abundant security cameras and possibly armed guards. Most have an initial entry, where staff checks your ID. You must enter and close the door behind you before proceeding. You must have a medical card to enter a medical dispensary. Many also require a driver's license or photo ID. Most states have minimum age requirements for entry.

Once your ID is checked, there is often another waiting room before you are invited into the dispensary proper. Review the menu and other promotional materials while you wait. If you have questions, ask for a patient care advocate. More experienced staff are usually available to sit down and answer your questions.

Buzz Words

Dispensary: A state-approved store where cannabis products are sold.

Bud Tender: Also known as a patient care advocate, a dispensary employee who works directly with customers to describe and sell cannabis products.

Exit Bag: In areas that require childproof packaging, exit bags childproof the order. Ask how they open.

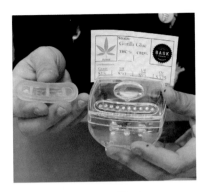

Photo: *Anna Meade*

Geek Out

Cannabis is sold in both grams and ounces.

Ounces to Grams

1/8	3.5
1/4	7
1/2	14
1	28

The sales area is typically well lit. A bud tender or patient care advocate (PCA) can describe their products and effects. They are usually very knowledgeable. Ask questions. The only bad question is the one you didn't ask.

Flower may be displayed in a sealed container. When the cap is lifted, you can smell the flower. You may be drawn to certain aromas. You can look at the flower, but generally, you do not handle it.

Some products are stored in glass cases with samples or written descriptions. Ask about cannabinoids and terpenes. Realize that some products may differ from the display.

Ask Your Bud Tender:

Tell them what effects you are seeking. Ask for products that have those effects. Ask if they tried the product and what they thought.

Flower: Where was it grown? Indoor or outdoor? Is it organic? Ask about pesticides used and lab test results.

Edibles: What is the strength? What is a single serving? What amount do new users typically consume?

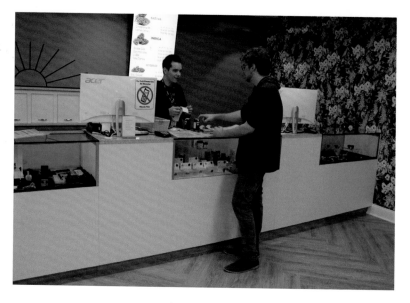

Photo: *Anna Meade*

Seven Tips for Shopping at a Dispensary

1. **Check the Website**: Lines and logistics, know before you go.
2. **Plan**: Consider why you want to use cannabis and what product(s) you want to try.
3. **Bring ID**: No ID, no entry.
4. **No Kids**: Leave them at home. No one under 21 is allowed.
5. **Bring Cash**: Dispensaries accept limited forms of payment.
6. **Security**: There are abundant security cameras and possibly armed guards.
7. **Wait**: Do not try your purchase in the parking lot or while driving your car.

Once you decide what you want, the cashier will ring your order. After you pay for it, it will be filled in the back. Double-check your order before leaving. Make sure you know how to open childproof containers and exit bags.

When you are leaving, the exit may be different than the entrance.

Do not light up in the parking lot. Consuming on site is not allowed. Some states require you to place the unopened bag in your trunk or glove compartment. You will have a better experience if you consume in a safe location with friends.

CANNABIS TOURISM

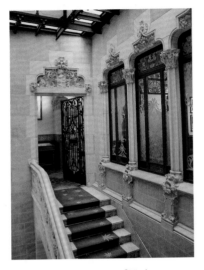

*Photo courtesy of Hash,
Marijuana & Hemp Museum*

Many people are visiting places where cannabis is legal so they can try it out. Canna-tourism has expanded beyond Amsterdam – from Jamaica to Canada and from California to Cape Cod.

However, rules vary and there are local restrictions. Smoking is restricted in most hotels. Find out the local laws before you travel so you can enjoy your trip without hassle. Understand that it is federally illegal in the US and TSA agents are federal officials whose main duty is airport security.

The Hash, Marijuana, & Hemp Museum of Barcelona is one of several beautiful museums that display artifacts of historical cannabis use. It is interesting to see how cannabis has been used around the world for generations.

Word to the Wise

You can buy CBD products in the gas station, chain stores and on-line. Buyers beware. Cannabis testing and regulation are still developing. Some products are not as advertised. Look for purity, independent testing, and reputable brands. Shop local and organic whenever possible.

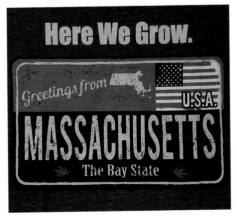

*Image use courtesy of Silver Screen
Designs / Photo: A. Sullivan*

CONSUMING CANNABIS

Finally, enjoying the herb. Set yourself up to have a nice experience. It is good to be in a comfortable place with friends.

Try cannabis in the evening. That way, if you have a bad experience, you can just sleep it off.

Try a very small amount at first. Some people do not feel anything the first time or the first few times they try cannabis. That is normal as your body adjusts. A day or two later, try a little more or less.

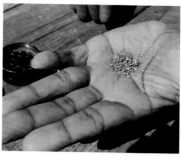

Photo courtesy of Trella Technologies, LLC

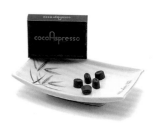

Photo: A. Sullivan

You may want to keep a journal while you discover how different products and amounts make you feel. There are sample journals in the appendix. You can also get journals at the dispensary or find an app.

Cannabis is evolving rapidly. As with any products, buyers beware. Different products will be available in various places, so choose wisely.

There are high and low quality products available. Some are tested and consistent. Others have no testing, are inconsistent, or have little value. Products from a licensed dispensary are typically tested and more consistent.

Cannabis flower can have mold or pesticides. Some CBD products are poor quality or have little or no CBD oils. There are also many great firms that bring quality products to market.

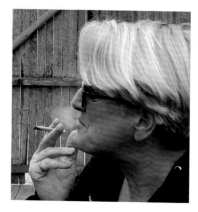

Photo: A. Sullivan

Tips for Your First Session

Relax and enjoy: Surround yourself with friends in a comfortable setting.

Time: Allow enough time for the possible effects. Make time in your schedule.

Low & slow: Try a small amount. Try more or less another evening.

Antidote: Have a CBD product or orange juice handy. They can calm you if too much THC makes you feel anxious.

You may build a tolerance for cannabis; more will be needed to have the same effect. You can reset your tolerance by taking a "tolerance break" and not consuming cannabis for 2-3 days.

This is only the beginning. You may start collecting beautiful glass pipes. You may infuse butter and make brownies for your friends. You may just take a pill before bedtime. Perhaps you will become an advocate or educator.

Wherever it leads, we hope you enjoy your cannabis journey. The end of prohibition is exciting. Many new products will be developed; some will have lasting value that will change our lives.

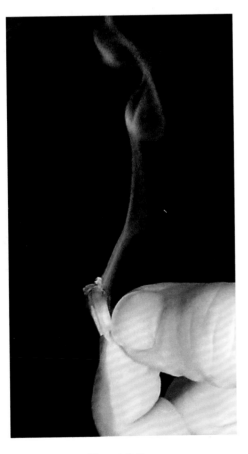

Photo: A. Sullivan

APPENDIX

There Are Two Main Cannabinoids In Cannabis:

THC
(Δ9-tetrahydrocannabinol)
psychoactive (euphoric high)
analgesic
anti-bacterial
anti-cancer
anti-inflammatory
anti-spasmodic
appetite stimulant
bone stimulant
bronchodilator
neuroprotective

CBD
(Cannabidiol)
non-euphoric, no high
analgesic
anti-anxiety
anti-bacterial
anti-cancer
anti-convulsive
anti-depressant
anti-emetic (anti-vomiting)
anti-inflammatory
anti-insomnia
anti-ischemic
(reverses reduced blood flow)
anti-psychotic
bone stimulant
immunosuppressive
neuroprotective

Image: Erica Giokas

Other Cannabinoids Found In Raw Cannabis:

CBG-A
(Cannabigerolic acid)
- analgesic
- anti-bacterial
- anti-cancer
- anti-depressant
- anti-fungal
- bone stimulant

CBG-A

THC-A
(Tetrahydrocannabinolic acid)
- anti-cancer
- anti-inflammatory
- anti-spasmodic

Δ⁹THC-A

CBD-A
(Cannabidiolic acid)
- anti-cancer
- anti-inflammatory

CBD-A

CBC-A
(Cannabichromenic acid)
- anti-inflammatory
- anti-fungal

CBC-A

Image: Erica Giokas

Other Cannabinoids Found In Cannabis After Heating Cannabis (Decarboxylation)

CBG
(Cannabigerol)

analgesic   anti-depressant
anti-bacterial   anti-fungal
anti-cancer   bone stimulant

CBG

CBGV
(Cannabigerivarin)
anti-convulsive
bone stimulant

CBGV

CBC
(Cannabichromene)

analgesic   anti-fungal
anti-bacterial   anti-inflammatory
anti-cancer   anti-insomnia
anti-depressant bone stimulant

CBC

THCV
(Tetrahydrocannabivarin)
anti-convulsive
anti-inflammatory
appetite suppressant
bone stimulant
neuroprotective

THCV

Image: Erica Giokas

Cannabinoid Synthesis

By simply applying heat or exposing cannabinoids to light and air there are a multitude of opportunities for other cannabinoids.

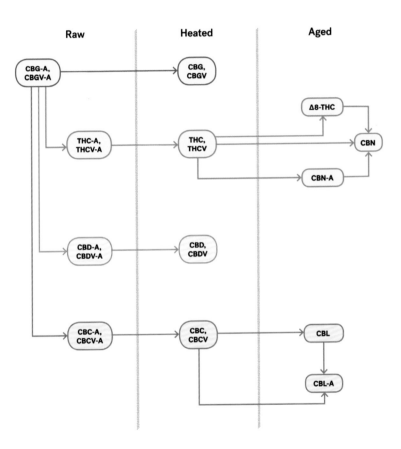

Image courtesy of Steep Hill Labs

THE

ENDOCANNABINOID SYSTEM

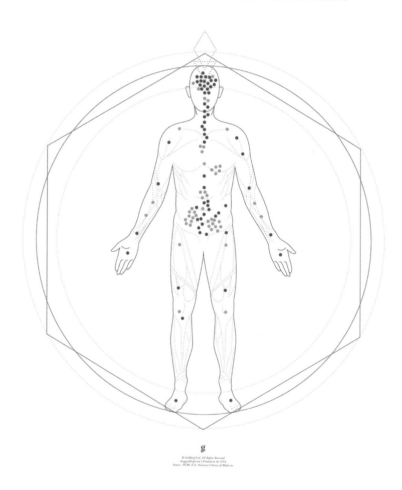

Image courtesy of Goldleaf

THE ENDOCANNABINOID SYSTEM

The human endocannabinoid system has two types of receptors that can uniquely receive the CBN, THC, and CBD molecules found in cannabis. The CB1 and CB2 receptors impact our physiological process affecting pain modulation, appetite, memory, anti-inflammatory response, and other immune system responses. These receptors are found on cell surfaces and although they are present in everyone, each body is different, which is why a wide range of reactions to these cannabinoids occur.

Although our bodies produce their own molecules that interact with the CB receptors (endogenous), molecules found in cannabis sativa (exogenous) are also perfectly engineered to interact with the same receptors.

- **CB1** Receives THC molecules. These receptors are concentrated in the brain, central nervous system and scattered throughout other bodily tissue. They mediate many of the psychoactive effects associated with cannabis.

- **CB2** Receives CBN molecules. These receptors are found in the peripheral organs and cells associated with the immune system and throughout the body. The highest concentration of these receptors is in the gut.

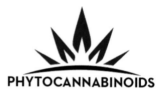

PHYTOCANNABINOIDS

	THC	CBD	CBG	CBN	CBC	THCV
Relieves Pain	●	●		●		
Reduces Seizures		●				●
Sedative				●		
Anti-anxiety		●				
Suppress Appetite			●			●
Anti-bacterial		●	●			
Anti-nausea	●	●				
Anti-fungal						
Inhibit Tumor Growth		●			●	
Anti-psychotic		●				
Suppress Muscle Spams	●	●				
Stimulate Appetite	●					
Anti-inflammatory		●	●		●	
Anti-insomnia		●			●	

wana

Image courtesy of Wana Brands

CANNABINOIDS

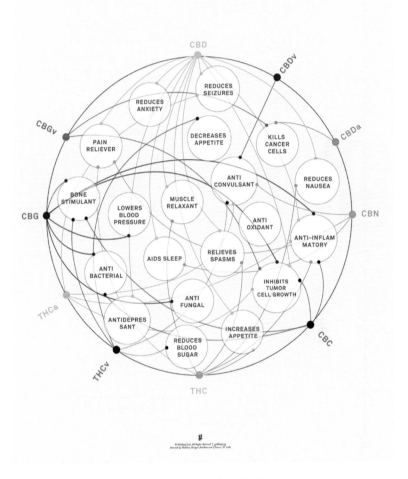

Image courtesy of Goldleaf

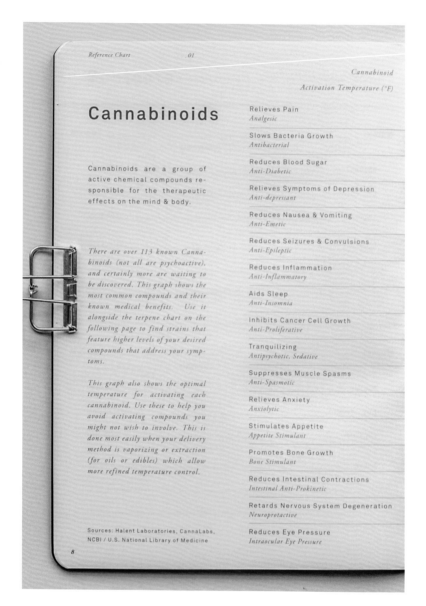

Cannabinoid

Activation Temperature (°F)

Cannabinoids

Cannabinoids are a group of active chemical compounds responsible for the therapeutic effects on the mind & body.

There are over 113 known Cannabinoids (not all are psychoactive), and certainly more are waiting to be discovered. This graph shows the most common compounds and their known medical benefits. Use it alongside the terpene chart on the following page to find strains that feature higher levels of your desired compounds that address your symptoms.

This graph also shows the optimal temperature for activating each cannabinoid. Use these to help you avoid activating compounds you might not wish to involve. This is done most easily when your delivery method is vaporizing or extraction (for oils or edibles) which allow more refined temperature control.

Sources: Halent Laboratories, CannaLabs, NCBI / U.S. National Library of Medicine

Relieves Pain
Analgesic

Slows Bacteria Growth
Antibacterial

Reduces Blood Sugar
Anti-Diabetic

Relieves Symptoms of Depression
Anti-depressant

Reduces Nausea & Vomiting
Anti-Emetic

Reduces Seizures & Convulsions
Anti-Epileptic

Reduces Inflammation
Anti-Inflammatory

Aids Sleep
Anti-Insomnia

Inhibits Cancer Cell Growth
Anti-Proliferative

Tranquilizing
Antipsychotic, Sedative

Suppresses Muscle Spasms
Anti-Spasmotic

Relieves Anxiety
Anxiolytic

Stimulates Appetite
Appetite Stimulant

Promotes Bone Growth
Bone Stimulant

Reduces Intestinal Contractions
Intestinal Anti-Prokinetic

Retards Nervous System Degeneration
Neuroprotactive

Reduces Eye Pressure
Intraocular Eye Pressure

8

Image courtesy of Goldleaf

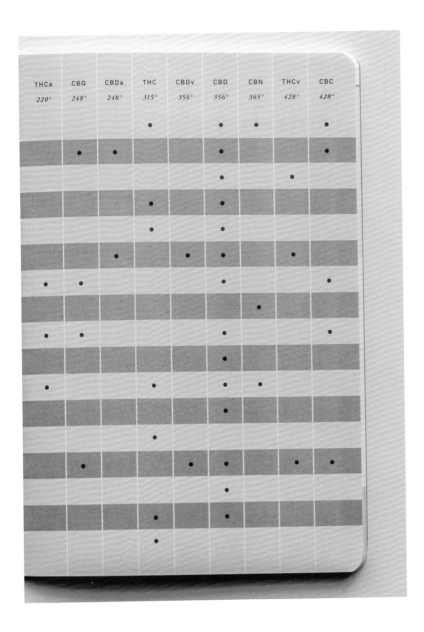

TERPENE PROFILES

The terpene profile of cannabis is complex. It takes a discerning nose and experience to be able to detect the nuances a specific cultivar possesses. Below is a visualization of different cannabis cultivars. Notice how different notes are depicted underneath stronger, more prominent smells.

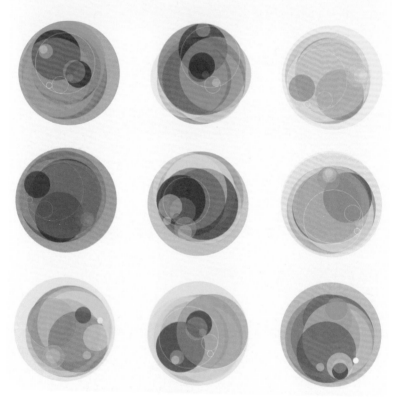

Image courtesy of Goldleaf

TRAIN YOUR NOSE

Most cannabis cultivars have one or two distinct notes. Often, these notes cover up the more subtle nuances contained in the terpene profile. Train your nose to be able to detect the other notes in a cultivar. What do you smell first? What else can you smell? The more you practice, the better you will become.

● **HUMULENE**
Boiling Point: 388°

● **CARYOPHYLLENE**
Boiling Point: 320°

● **VALENCENE**
Boiling Point: 253°

● **MYRCENE**
Boiling Point: 334°

● **TERPINOLENE**
Boiling Point: 220°

● **BISABOLOL**
Boiling Point: 307°

● **LINALOOL**
Boiling Point: 388°

● **PINENE**
Boiling Point: 311°

● **OCIMENE**
Boiling Point: 122°

● **TERPINEOL**
Boiling Point: 423°

● **GERANIOL**
Boiling Point: 446°

● **LIMONENE**
Boiling Point: 349°

g

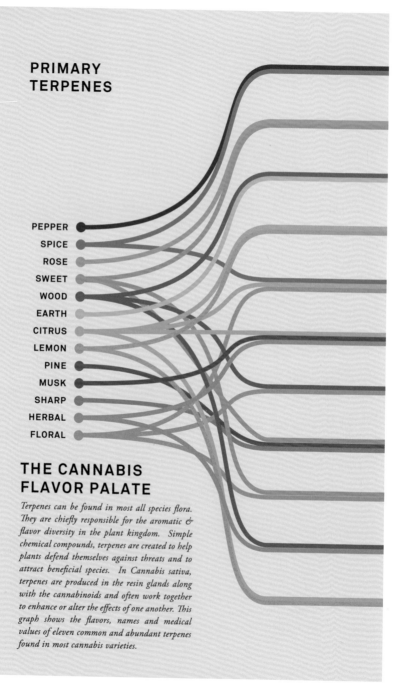

**PRIMARY
TERPENES**

PEPPER
SPICE
ROSE
SWEET
WOOD
EARTH
CITRUS
LEMON
PINE
MUSK
SHARP
HERBAL
FLORAL

THE CANNABIS
FLAVOR PALATE

Terpenes can be found in most all species flora. They are chiefly responsible for the aromatic & flavor diversity in the plant kingdom. Simple chemical compounds, terpenes are created to help plants defend themselves against threats and to attract beneficial species. In Cannabis sativa, terpenes are produced in the resin glands along with the cannabinoids and often work together to enhance or alter the effects of one another. This graph shows the flavors, names and medical values of eleven common and abundant terpenes found in most cannabis varieties.

Image courtesy of Goldleaf

Appendix

CARYOPHYLLENE
Known to have an aroma that is peppery, woody, and spicy, this is the only terpene proven to interact with the endocannabinoid system (CB2) in our bodies. It is also found in basil, oregano, pepper, and cinnamon.
Medical value: anti-inflammatory, analgesic, anti-spasmodic, sleep aid

GERANIOL
Creating a delightfully sweet smell akin to roses, this terpene is present in geraniums, lemons, and tobacco and is often used in perfumes and other cosmetics. It is also an effective mosquito repellent.
Medical value: Neuroprotective, anti-fungal, anti-tumor

HUMULENE
Another strong contributor to the tell-tale "earthy" aroma of cannabis, this terpene is also present in hops and coriander. Humulene can act as an appetite suppressant and offers potent anti-inflammatory abilities.
Medical value: anti-inflammatory, antibacterial, analgesic

LIMOLENE
Common in sativa varieties, it is associated with elevated mood. It can also be found in citrus rinds, juniper, and mint. Limonene has a unique ability to quicken the absorption of other terpenes in the body.
Medical value: antixiolytic, anti-depressant, gastroesophageal reflux, and anti-fungal

LINALOOL
This terpene's hallmark is its floral scent, reminiscent of sharp and sweet wildflowers. It is also found in lavender, laurel, birch, and rosewood. It has calming and sedative properties and can help relieve anxiety.
Medical value: analgesic, anti-epileptic, anti-depressant

MYRCENE
Described as earthy and musky, this terpene is prevalent in most all of the strains of cannabis and is known to enhance THC uptake in the body. Myrcene is also found in mango, hops, thyme, and citrus.
Medical value: analgesic, anti-inflammatory, antibacterial, sedative

OCIMENE
Found in a wide variety of botanicals, it is known for its sweet and woody scent. Plants use ocimene to defend themselves against pests in nature. It is also found in mint, parsley, pepper, basil, orchids, and kumquats.
Medical value: antifungal

PINENE
The most common naturally occurring terpene, it is a main contributor to cannabis' tell-tale piney aroma. It is also found in many conifer species and herbs such as sage. It is known to enhance memory and alertness.
Medical value: anti-inflammatory, bronchodilator

TERPINEOL
Due to its pleasant aroma, reminiscent of lilac flower blossoms, it is often used in cosmetic products. It is often found in higher concentrations alongside of pinene which unfortunately may mask its scent.
Medical value: antibacterial, anti-anxiety, immunostimulant.

TERPINOLENE
Having a piney aroma with notes of herbs and wildflowers, this terpene is a useful insect repellent. It is also found in rosemary, sage and cypress. Terpinolene has been shown to exhibit anticancer and tranquilizing effects.
Medical value: sedative, and anti-proliferative.

VALENCENE
With a citrusy sweet aroma, this terpene is also found in grapefruits, tangerines, oranges, and some herbs. It is common in many strains of cannabis and is shown to be a powerful tick and mosquito repellent.
*Medical value: *still being researched*

Report of Sample Analysis

Cannabiz
(555) 555 0420
qcpro@cbf.com

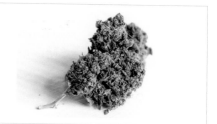

Sample Name:	Chemdog
Sample type:	Flower
Batch/Project:	N/A
Product ID:	S17xxx-0710
Receipt Date:	04/20/2018
Test Date:	04/22/2018
Total Analytes:	30.08%

Cannabinoid Profile

■ THCa	21.5%
■ CBDa	1.6%
■ CBGa	1.7%
■ THC	1.2%
■ CBD	0.1%
▫ CBN	<0.1%
■ Δ–8THC	<0.1%
■ THCv	<0.1%
■ CBDv	<0.1%
■ CBC	<0.1%
Total Cannabinoids	26.1%
Max THC	20.06%
Max CBD	1.5%

Terpene Profile

■ β-Caryophyllene	0.96%
■ Nerolidol 2	0.92%
■ β-Myrcene	0.86%
■ α-Humulene	0.44%
▫ Ocimene	0.19%
■ α-Pinene	0.18%
■ β-Pinene	0.11%
■ Linalool	0.07%
▫ Caryophyllene Oxide	0.06%
■ Isopulegol	0.05%
■ Camphene	0.05%
■ β-Ocimene	0.03%
■ Terpinolene	0.03%
■ Nerolidol 1	0.02%
■ γ-Terpinene	0.01%
▫ δ-3-Carene	<0.01%
▫ α-Terpinene	<0.01%
▫ δ-Limonene	<0.01%
▫ Eucalyptol	<0.01%
▫ Geraniol	<0.01%
▫ Guaiol	<0.01%
▫ α-Bisabolol	<0.01%
Total Terpenes	3.98%

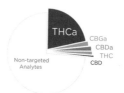

THCa is converted to THC by heat. Use the following formula to find the **max THC**:

Max THC = THC + (THCa x **0.877**).

CBDa is converted to CBD by heat. Use the following formula to find the **max CBD**:

Max CBD = CBD + (CBDa x **0.877**).

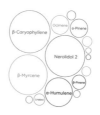

Disclaimer: Data represents weight of sample as received by MCR Labs. bubble graph represents amount of terpene in sample compared only to other detected terpenes.

85 Speen Street
Framingham, MA 01701
508 872 6666
www.mcrlabs.com

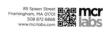

Image courtesy of MCR Labs

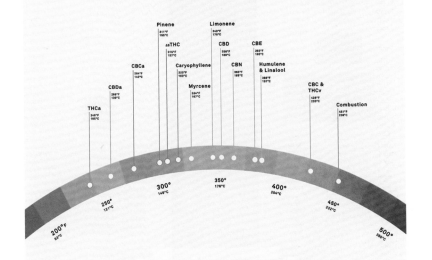

ACTIVATION TEMPERATURE

The boiling point of various chemical compounds found in cannabis.

This chart shows the most common cannabinoids & terpenes found in cannabis, as well as their known temperature for activation. This temperature is the point at which solids become gas, and chemical metamorphosis takes place. By heating to the specified level or just above, you ensure maximum efficacy of the compound listed, and reduce the likelihood of activating other compounds you might not wish to consume.

Image courtesy of Goldleaf

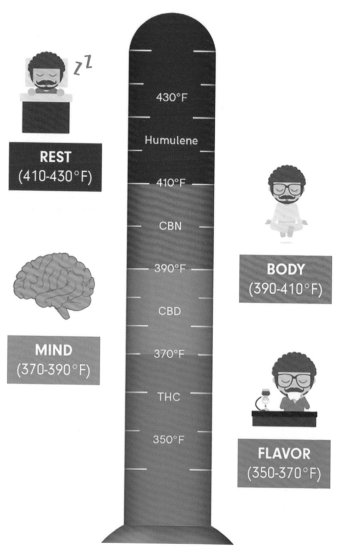

DAVINCI
WHAT'S YOUR PATH?

REST
(410-430°F)

430°F

Humulene

410°F

CBN

390°F

CBD

370°F

THC

350°F

BODY
(390-410°F)

MIND
(370-390°F)

FLAVOR
(350-370°F)

Image courtesy of Davinci

CANNABIS TEMP GUIDE

THC (315°F) - Cannabinoid - Strongly psychoactive (gets you high), helps treat pain, nausea, sleep and stress disorders, and appetite loss. Can also cause anxiety and paranoia.

Myrcene (345°F) - Terpene - Also found in mangos, hops, and lemongrass. Gives a sedating or relaxing effect. Actually increases THC's psychoactivity.

Limonene (349°F) - Terpene - Bitter citrus aroma, also found in fruit rinds and peppermint. Helps treat gastric reflux, fungus, depression, and anxiety.

CBD (350°F) - Cannabinoid - Non-psychoactive (no euphoric high). Gives a calming effect and helps treat anxiety, sleep loss, pain, multiple sclerosis, inflammation, stress, and epilepsy.

CBN (365°F) - Cannabinoid - Mildly psychoactive (does not include euphoric high) typically only occurs as a result of THC degradation. Helps treat insomnia, glaucoma, and pain.

Humulene (380°F) - Terpene - Aroma similar to hops. Has anti-bacterial and anti-inflammatory properties. Actually helps diminish your appetite or combat the munchies.

Linalool (390°F) - Terpene - Floral aroma, also found in lavender has anti-insomnia, anti-psychotic, anti-epileptic, anti-anxiety, and painkilling properties.

CBC (428°F) - Cannabinoid - Non-psychoactive (does not induce a euphoric high). 10 times more effective than CBD in treating anxiety and stress anti-inflammatory and anti-viral properties.

Image courtesy of Davinci

Date	Time	Product	Method Of Consumption (Inhale, Ingest, Etc)	Amount	Effects

Cannabis Consumption Journal

Record your purchases and consumption experiences.

Purchase: What did you buy, from where, when?

Product: _____ Amount: _____
Purchased from: _____ On: _____
Notes: (smell, freshness, color, cannabinoid and terpene profile)

Consumption Experience #1
Consumption? Duration? Effects?

I consumed (amount, when, where, who with) _____
Duration: kicked in: _____ wore off: _____
How did you feel before and after?

Consumption Experience #2
Consumption? Duration? Effects?

I consumed (amount, when, where, who with) _____
Duration: kicked in: _____ wore off: _____
How did you feel before and after?

Consumption Experience #3
Consumption? Duration? Effects?

I consumed (amount, when, where, who with) _____
Duration: kicked in:_____ wore off: _____
How did you feel before and after?

Cannabis Consumption Journal

Record your purchases and consumption experiences.

Purchase: What did you buy, from where, when?

Product: _____ Amount: _____
Purchased from: _____ On: _____
Notes: (smell, freshness, color, cannabinoid and terpene profile)

Consumption Experience #1
Consumption? Duration? Effects?

I consumed (amount, when, where, who with) _____
Duration: kicked in: _____ wore off: _____
How did you feel before and after?

Consumption Experience #2
Consumption? Duration? Effects?

I consumed (amount, when, where, who with) _____
Duration: kicked in: _____ wore off: _____
How did you feel before and after?

Consumption Experience #3
Consumption? Duration? Effects?

I consumed (amount, when, where, who with) _____
Duration: kicked in:_____ wore off: _____
How did you feel before and after?

Cannabis Consumption Journal

Record your purchases and consumption experiences.

Purchase: What did you buy, from where, when?

Product: _____ Amount: _____

Purchased from: _____ On: _____

Notes: (smell, freshness, color, cannabinoid and terpene profile)

Consumption Experience #1
Consumption? Duration? Effects?

I consumed (amount, when, where, who with) _____

Duration: kicked in: _____ wore off: _____

How did you feel before and after?

Consumption Experience #2
Consumption? Duration? Effects?

I consumed (amount, when, where, who with) _____

Duration: kicked in: _____ wore off: _____

How did you feel before and after?

Consumption Experience #3
Consumption? Duration? Effects?

I consumed (amount, when, where, who with) _____

Duration: kicked in:_____ wore off: _____

How did you feel before and after?

Cannabis Consumption Journal

Record your purchases and consumption experiences.

Purchase: What did you buy, from where, when?

Product: _____ Amount: _____
Purchased from: _____ On: _____
Notes: (smell, freshness, color, cannabinoid and terpene profile)

Consumption Experience #1
Consumption? Duration? Effects?

I consumed (amount, when, where, who with) _____
Duration: kicked in: _____ wore off: _____
How did you feel before and after?

Consumption Experience #2
Consumption? Duration? Effects?

I consumed (amount, when, where, who with) _____
Duration: kicked in: _____ wore off: _____
How did you feel before and after?

Consumption Experience #3
Consumption? Duration? Effects?

I consumed (amount, when, where, who with) _____
Duration: kicked in:_____ wore off: _____
How did you feel before and after?

NOTES

NOTES